MEN AT BIRTH

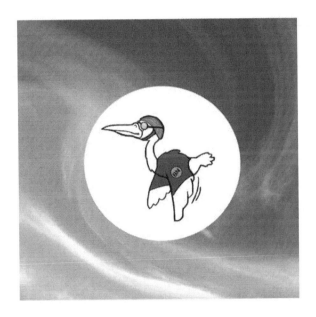

Guide to a Successful Childbirth

Phillip and Genny White
Birth Navigators
© 2009

Summer 2009
Navigate Press
Orange, CA

Copyright © 2009 by Phillip and Genny White

ISBN: 978-1442126756

1. Pregnancy—Popular works.
2. Childbirth—Popular works.
3. Fathers
4. Husbands

White, Genny 1965
White, Phillip B. 1961
Men at Birth: Guide to a Successful Childbirth Experience
Phil & Genny White

1st Ed.
Back cover photo: Jim Johnson Custom Photography, GR8FOTO.com

Table of Contents

CHAPTER 16: DEALING WITH THE UNEXPECTED 182

CHAPTER 17: THE WAYS OF NATURAL CHILDBIRTH 192

CHAPTER 18: AFTER THE LANDING 201

APPENDIX A: INTERVIEWING A PHYSICIAN 210

Acknowledgements

We would like to thank all of those who supported us in putting this together. Appreciation goes out to Dr. and Mrs. William Sears who met with us for dinner to discuss the book idea. Thank you Mr. Scott Dunphy for the encouragement and humor and for reviewing advanced copies. Seattle Midwifery School was significant in teaching us about the whole realm of childbirth in America. Dr. Mary Ann Armenteros was a major help by believing in natural childbirth as a choice and midwifery as a solution. It is often said that when the pupil is ready the teacher shall appear, and for Genny that could not be truer. We wish to express our gratitude to Genny's foremost teacher and mentor Karen Baker, LM. Karen has made in surmountable contributions both to the worlds of midwifery and midwifery education. She is both a sterling midwife and an exemplary teacher of midwives. Karen, thank you for all the lessons you taught. Our family deserves praise for putting up with us and learning more about birth than kids should know at any age, thank you Julia, Corban, Jacob, and Isaiah White. To Joanne Myers-Ciecko thanks for providing information relevant to the topic and to Leslie Butterfield for being an inspiration and mentor. We would like to thank Patty Brumbaugh, CNM posthumous for her visionary work in midwifery and for all she meant to us personally as well as to others in her pioneering work in facilitating and assisting families to have vaginal births after a previous cesarean experience. We would like to thank Dr. James and Cathy Brodsky for all their tireless work to improve the health and healthcare in our community. We would like to say thank you to Gwen Wessells, whose passion for nutritional excellence is both contagious and inspiring. Also we would like to thank Therese Charvet for her leadership and professionalism by role modeling equity and tolerance. We express gratitude to all the authors of all the books from which we read and studied as you paved the way for us and opened our heart and minds to the need for men to be better educated on the topic.

Introduction

This book is designed to help you learn how to assist your mate in the course of pregnancy and childbirth. Knowledge is power, and many men are not properly trained or experienced enough to know what this experience is really like. For many guys, childbirth can be a scary and stressful event. We hope to enlighten you, to empower you and to prepare you for what may be coming.

Childbirth can be a major frustration for men since they are not experiencing it directly. It is also not a problem that men can solve. However, you may find like Phil did that childbirth is a personal trial. In this book we use the analogy that you are the wingman, flying a mission to protect the success of the flight. Your job is to know what the primary pilot needs, to understand the inherent dangers of the journey, and to be support when called upon. For some, connecting the idea that birth could be related to warfare is a stretch, but psychologically men want to take the role of protectors, but they are ill-equipped to handle childbirth without training. That is why we hope you will read this book. We want you to ask questions, we want to help you through this basic training.

You may have questions that go unanswered after you read this book, and we will try to make it possible for you to contact us through the internet. We can be contacted online at **www.birthnavigators.com.** We would like to hear from you about whether you liked our book and about how your pregnancy and childbirth experience went. Photos and birth stories are welcomed, too.

Birth can be one of the best moments in your life, and we want you to experience the joys and satisfactions that childbirth can give personally. There is no guarantee of that, but without plans, one basically plans to fail. Your taking the time to be involved especially in the planning can help to solidify your relationship with your partner and coming child.

We would like to walk along side you by providing information from our experience and readings that have relevance to what men need to know about birth. We have started calling ourselves Birth Navigators because we have been through this challenging experience four times. You too will soon need to navigate a childbirth experience on your own. By reading this book we hope to open your mind to how you can be of practical and emotional support to your mate.

Introduction to Health Care Professionals
Why This Book is Necessary

I am writing this to my fellow peers. Over the years I have enjoyed the rich opportunity of exchanging ideas and information with you through the course of my education and training opportunities. In these training exercises and in services with the people who care for our country's childbearing families, midwifes, women's health care and obstetrical nurses, Doulas, professional labor support providers and childbirth educators one can almost discern a palpable pulse of sorority a common bond of commitment to the cause of contributing our personal best to assist the childbearing community to have safe satisfying birth experiences. It is to you that I address this introduction; why this book is necessary? Our literature is extensive with child birth education materials. There are many titles that can come immediately to our minds. Our market is saturated with bright glossy childbirth education information produced and provided by the industries that profit from new parents diapers and formula companies.

Why do we need another childbirth education tool? All of our present childbirth education culture is not specifically geared to speak to the fathers, to the men in our country. I believe that if men understand what is at stake for themselves and in the lives of the women and children that they care for throughout a childbirth experience that they will become more attentive and proactive in how birth occurs in their own families, and in their communities and perhaps eventually there will be a male voice advocating for reforms and normalcy in the American childbirth experience. In the words of Agnes Sallet Von Tannenberg, "If we are to heal the planet, we must begin by healing birthing."

We need the male voice to call for the healing of birth also. Men are wired differently from women, and we have attempted to communicate to men in their unique style of communication what is exactly at stake in their childbirth experience. And is there a time or season in a couple's life that demands more clear communication than that of the childbearing season? Dr. John Gray introduces us to his land breaking book <u>Men Are From Mars, Women Are From Venus</u> on how the sexes communicate differently by revisiting with us a postpartum experience between his wife and himself.

The season of childbirth is so heightened and is so influential we cannot afford to disregard the differences between the way the sexes communicate, and it is time for men to have a means of understanding the sacred women's experience of childbirth. At first it may seem foreign to envision stealthy cold steel fighter jets as tools to illustrate the woman centered nature of childbirth, even antithetical to see emblems of the male establishment of war and defense representing what we understand to be as natural as a warm and cozy parlor set up for tea or a girls' sleep over, but if a flash of a flight jacket and the correlations between childbirth and flying sorties will be a tool that enables men to grasp just how important childbirth is to all of society, these tools should be used and used quickly in the education of men about childbirth. To not see and respect the differences in the way the sexes communicate and to not make allowances to the male species is to be sexist. For those of you who may scoff at this idea, I challenge you to realize that we are trying to communicate in a way that the people you care about need to hear the message. We are speaking to your brothers, your lovers, maybe even your sons and if the tool we provide them with serves to give them a grasp to the reality of childbirth then maybe we can begin to truly see inroads to quality health care for childbearing families in our country.

Genny White
August 6, 2009
Orange, CA

Biography

Phillip and Genny White met in college in the 1980's and were married in 1984, the year Phillip graduated from East Carolina University with a BA in English. They traveled to Boston where Phillip obtained a Master's in Professional Writing from Emerson College in 1989. Genny studied at Seattle Midwifery School for three years in the early 2000s.

The two have four children. They have experienced a wide range of birth experiences, from a traumatic emergency cesarean to a home birth. Their first child was delivered after an emergency cesarean. They navigated the emotional obstacle course of accomplishing their next birth, a successful, Midwife-attended VBAC, in a hospital.

Three years later they celebrated their third birth, a water birth, attended by midwives in a freestanding birth center. This water birth was the first water birth at that birth center. Not only was this a fulfilling vaginal birth after a previous cesarean. Phillip and Genny's dream of having these maternity health benefits covered by an insurance carrier was realized. After consistent petitioning, their insurance provider (Blue Cross) paid the freestanding birth center for the birth. This event paved the way for other families to be able to access the birth option of a freestanding birth center. In 1997, after a Midwife-attended home birth, the couple welcomed their fourth child into their family.

After experiencing their traumatic first experience, they continued adding to their knowledge base during the other pregnancies while exploring, researching, and empowering themselves to bring to fruition an environment conducive to having a vaginal birth after a cesarean. The discoveries they made ignited the desire to shed a light in the darkness of how contemporary society manages birth.

Phillip's personal experiences galvanized him to want to be a voice to men facing the unknown of childbirth. He feels that men need to pick back up the traditional role of providing protection to their partners during the vulnerable time of pregnancy, birth and the postpartum period. Many men feel impotent concerning their roles in the bearing of children. Little formal or societal training exists, leaving men powerless and ignorant. Fathers feel quite intimidated when trying to fend off the medical establishment, and they can be emotionally overwhelmed when attending a birth. He hopes that men reading this book will be able to protect their partners from often unnecessary but standardized medical protocols and procedures and from negative birth experiences and also that they will learn their true place in the childbirth experience.

Preface: Why Family Matters

The building blocks of any healthy society are families. The basic core of all human civilizations is this integral unit. The framework of government, establishment of law, structure of human existence is in the establishment of strong, vibrant and vigorous families.

Try to picture men as empty steel one-dimensional boxes. Lined next to each other you just have more of a blue print than a structure. Men without women are like unpainted or unfinished. They have little flair and no comprehension of the richness of life. Add in a dash of love for a woman, and they light up. They change from directionless and self-absorbed creatures who have no interest in the betterment of mankind into men of purpose, who are focused and productive.

Women are the knitters of society. They create the community, the connection from one box to another. So men without women are consumers of the good of society and men with women begin becoming producers for the growth and health of society.

This is magnified exponentially when a child is born. The child stretches the couple to create another dimension of societal value. It is like the square with color now is a cube.

All this is opposed to narcissistic, selfish form of existence that is immature. Most men grow out of their self focused lifestyles when they get married. They learn new forms of love and take on new duties and responsibilities. That is what is absolutely needed for society to be healthy.

The whole of society should be about developing a healthy place for children to be raised and nurtured. A healthy society will impose law and order to protect the family and ensure the health of the family.

Men really need to get a clue. Sex can result in pregnancy; it isn't all about having pleasure. If men aren't willing to take on the responsibility of being a parent, then men are risking tearing holes in the fabric of human society. Reckless self centered living is always damaging to others. All the familiar negative cultural problems relate to this: drugs, crime, pornography, alcoholism, gambling. When people are caught up in self pleasuring, they are harming themselves, others, and society.

Men become men when they get out of themselves and learn to live for others – that is mature satisfaction. When they place the safety and concern of others ahead of their own pleasures, they are real men. That is what family provides men: a reason to be men. Men need family to be men.

Take warfare. What motivates men the most is when they are protecting their family, the neighbors, and their society from others who have come to destroy it. The defense of a healthy society is what made America so great in World War II. Men willingly signed up to fight that war. That was not the case in Vietnam, men were forced. They were not defending their families, their culture nor their society.

So when a male fathers a child, that is the beginning of greatness, of building a greater America, and a greater world. How much more purpose and how much more can a man be a man then to fill their little cube with a family? Having children creates a higher level of love and provides the connections to a reason for creating a healthy society, government and world. Ultimately the family changes males to men, providing them the purpose and desire to perform duties and responsibilities beyond those that only satisfy their base appetites. Without a family men are without reason for performing those duties, or caring about their society and culture. They only care about themselves. Raising a family one of the highest purposes in life and provides reason for all men do.

Phillip White
August 6, 2009
Orange, CA

Chapter 1: First Briefing

Congratulations Are In Order

Welcome gentlemen, this is your first briefing with Birth Navigators. Today you are to be congratulated on beginning your mission to fatherhood. The course you are on will lead you to many new and exciting developments in your life. This is a road the whole of humanity has traveled since the beginning of time. With something as momentous and astounding as the creation of another human, we should all be popping open some champagne and toasting each father reading this. Yet, that can wait until the mission is completed and everyone arrives home safe and sound.

First of all let's consider what your child will mean to you in the global sense. Each of us has a definitive time of live on this earth. By producing offspring, we ensure that part of us moves on to the next generation. We are all here by this process, and we have joined the ranks of millions upon millions of other fathers. This community is as diverse as the faces making it up. Anyone with a little spiritual insight can see that birth is the essence of life, both biologically and physically. Bringing life and order is the genius of humanity. When you have a child coming, think of it as the greatest gift you can receive. A good father plans a life of order, discipline and love for that coming child.

What is this child going to mean to you? If you have a boy, is this going to be your best buddy in the world? If it is a girl, has the beautiful princess of your life arrived? Our imaginations are not capable of perceiving the reality of what a newborn child can bring. The expressions of all of us with children are only faint glimpses of what it truly can mean for you. Savor the experience and enjoy it with your whole being. Some joys cannot be shared or eluded to. One must receive the joyous reward privately.

Now that we have celebrated fatherhood, we need to move on to the ramifications of the coming months. A new child brings about a myriad of changes, and for many, change is unwelcome. Buckle your belt and be prepared for alterations in your life!

Your Promotion

You have a short time to prepare for the arrival of this new life, this gift of life. This is time that needs to be well spent and you need to get to work as soon as possible. Time stops for no one. Let's reflect on what is coming, along with the baby. First, there is your relationship with the mother to be. Then you have the commitments required to establish a home for a child. There are also the physiological changes your partner is going to be going through. Next you may have financial concerns to think about. You may also have a plethora of other issues like in-laws, other children, and other important relationships that will be affected. A coming child and a pregnancy will change life as you have known it. You have a new assignment with new responsibilities. Birth is a test of human character, so schedule some time to learn everything you can to pass the exam with flying colors. You have a new assignment now. Yes, you have been promoted! You have a new mission.

The Unknown

Here we are, observing the murky crystal ball, feeling the phantom future's stirrings, or listening for the prophet's whisperings. Though we may not perceive these portents, we are not without power. We must find our place in birth. We must stand up and be the men that we are. Yet, we need direction. We need our own vision, our own rhythm and harmony. Where do we stand? When the music starts, how do we dance? For most of us, this unknown is a bit intimidating. We don't carry the child. We don't push. We don't frankly know what to do. Most of us would rather disconnect. We'd rather watch the World Series, a hockey game, check the markets, or go to work. This touchy feely thing is not our bag and men know it.

Some teachings and some childbirth educators would have us be the birth coach, and some of us may manage to be there in that capacity, but birth takes us into foreign territory, and without a clear cut understanding of what the heck you are to do at a birth and what your place is, you will have all those feelings of awkwardness. So let's uncover who you are and what you can do to be involved in this process of pregnancy and childbirth.

Becoming a Birth Navigator

This message is to strengthen your resolve, to provide you with intelligence, and to give you the best advice to help you become the best navigator for your child's entrance into this world. Your partner did not get to this place without you, and she shouldn't have to fly this mission alone. Once you choose to make the commitment to being involved, you are part of the birth team.

The reason we have chosen to use the analogy of flying a military mission is that delivering a baby can become a dangerous journey. First, your partner and your baby are at risk. The way birth is handled in North America adds to the dangers. So you need to be ready to protect your family. Though there have been advances in medicine in the last century, in the last thirty to forty years birth has not become any safer for women and children. While technology has replaced the human touch in birth, mortality rates have stayed the same, so is the technology helping? As the Top Gun training center was created to retrain fighter pilots in the art of dog fighting because pilots had been relying too much on the technology and getting shot down, we believe Americans need to learn again how to birth.

You need to learn about the dangers, and to take your role of protector seriously. There are a variety of negative outcomes, some of which you can do nothing to avoid, but there are others which are unnecessary and are avoidable. All negative outcomes will impact your relationship with your partner; some will even end that relationship, so you must do everything in your power to be prepared for birth.

When there are serious complications in childbirth, especially those not prepared for, there are dire consequences. The vast majority of births that end in the death of the baby will cause the couple to divorce or separate. Some say that about eighty percent of births that end with an unexpected emergency surgery break up. So if you value your relationship, you are going to have to take this thing seriously. Protect your interests and do everything you can to avoid a bad outcome. The more you know the better you will be able to protect your forming family.

Preparing for Take Off

Sexual love can be a base thing or a holy sanctified act. It can be a divine experience or a sadistic vile act of hatred. If you are reading this book, you've probably have established a relationship with your partner that has deeper roots of strength than just a passing physical relationship. Yet passion can produce more than pleasure, it can produce beauty beyond compare. Do not be afraid to touch the hand of the creator, for that hand has already been close by. The miracle of life is never more visible then when you hold in your hands the child of your union.

Physical, sexual love is like taking a powerful F15 fighter up into the air. The acceleration and the joy of 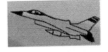 physical intercourse is as powerful as any other physical act and has the same high, the same crescendo. Intercourse does not always bring conception of a child. Of course, the woman's reproductive system in many ways represents the flower blossoming. Everything about the woman is in running a cycle of preparing for this joyous explosion of love. And everything about the pleasure of planting that seed is explosive. But, once the conception occurs, the woman's body unalterably changes. They say that the cells of a baby actually alter the woman's chemistry indefinitely, and that the child's cells remain inside the woman for years. No one is sure exactly how this affects a pregnant woman, but it is fascinating. This biochemical force alters the very state of a woman. The deep-seated nurturing nature of a mother is a quality that has secured man from the brink of death and extinction for eons.

You may have read that a woman protects her children like a she-bear protects its young. You don't want to mess with a woman's kids. Women don't do a lot of killing, but injure her young, and you may find out what a bear is like. You read about that essence in stories depicting mothers whose child was killed by a drunk driver, or abducted or through some other horrific act of violence or injustice.

At birth, now here is the very moment where the bear is physically unable to come to her cub's defense. She is at her most vulnerable. She needs someone to stand up for her and to protect her while she is in the throes of labor. As the baby is undergoing a tense passage through the birth canal, twisting and turning, both mother and child are simultaneously being stressed. If it is your partner's first birth, her whole carriage has to loosen up, her hips spread apart, and her body open like never before. This strain on her body is nothing compared to the mental angst. Women describe it as having to give up total control of their body for a time and that can be a crushing feeling. We men merely stand around watching, feeling helpless ourselves to do anything. We may be informed and supportive, but we can do nothing that feels like we can fix labor. We suspect that is why the medical establishment has imposed so many interventions. They are trying to do something, but it is best just to overcome that feeling of trying to fix our partner's and letting nature run its course.

What we can do is to comfort and support our partners, caressing their hair, massaging their backs, and holding the drink cup. This is an emotional time for men, and one that shouldn't be taken lightly. More importantly, knowing that we make a difference before the birth is the best way of ensuring a safe environment with a quality birth team.

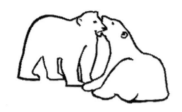

We find it incredibly amazing how in nature polar bears deal with birth. The male, the father bear, leaves the females and the mother to the birth. He distances himself at say a mile radius. Then as the birth is happening, that big old poppa bear aggressively defends that territory. Nothing enters that circle: caribou, other bears, human beings, whatever; they are in his sights. He will kill anything that encroaches upon the birth. Birth is to be protected with life and limb.

Where does that leave us men, after a child is conceived? Most men after this point are at a loss, out of their comfort zone. They didn't need a manual for the exhilaration of the sexual union, yet conception and pregnancy alters the relationship between lovers. The woman now has this cargo aboard. Never again will the relationship be the same. The free flying days are now like our exhaust trails. Men find they don't know what to say, what to do and how to act once the baby comes into the picture.

Change of Missions

Let's say that the mission of the sexual union was to provide exhilarating physical and emotional bonding between man and woman. Now what do you suppose the mission is when there is a child on its way? Could it be the same? But just at a more intensified level?

Some people chose to eject and bale out. But, you, Sir, obviously have chosen to commit to the mission. The commitment in becoming a father is crucial. You must have the courage to learn your place in pregnancy and birth – what you learn will prepare your character for fatherhood.

Experience declares the mother is the captain of the mission. You are the wingman. The baby is growing in her, changing her role in life. Her nature shifts dramatically. Her priorities will rearrange as she prepares for the birth. It is not just her body that changes; her diet, her habits and her preferences all amend. As an old proverb says, "How can two walk together unless they walk in agreement?" For you to fly along side of your partner, you have got to keep attention and watch her plane. You've got to be focused in on her and perceiving these modifications. You need to encourage her and support her in all that is transpiring.

Most women will admit to each other that every pregnancy has fear. Part of your work is to learn how to help her overcome that fear – usually directed at the unknown since each birth is different from any other. The more knowledge you have the better your ability to adjust the plane as it flies along. If you have ever seen an air show, you have already marveled at the way the planes stay in tight formations, and then perform aerobatic marvels. Well, pregnancy and birth are themselves dances that need serious planning and communication. When all goes well, you will have gained a great deal in your relationship. Your partner will grow to trust, respect and admire you as you hold her hand through the process that brings new life.

Yet, when you get to the birthing hour, the woman is not controlling the birth, her body is. Some say the uterus is truly in control. But the environment where the birth occurs is a huge factor in how the mission will turn out. That is why even the best-intentioned father may find that his presence can offset all the negative environmental factors. The choice of environments in which to have a birth is something men can have a whole lot to do with. Mark your territory. Set your sights on the new mission.

Conclusion

This ends our first briefing. The seed is planted, and you must do everything in your power to ensure that that seed is nurtured and grows well. You realize that you can only do so much, but what you do matters. Your primary responsibility is to be the protector of your partner and child. Think about it. Fatherhood has the most significant requirements placing on you important responsibilities, and at the same time it can be the biggest joys of your life, and can expand the amount of love and pleasure you experience. Imagine a good future, and be committed to ensuring that by your actions, attentions and attitudes, and you can expect nothing but positive results. Take responsibility for your place as father and lover.

Chapter 2: The New Mission

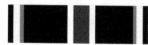

The Vision

Can you visualize what this pregnancy and birth are going to be like? Have you been through one of these missions before? Well, no matter what you visualize, every birth is a separate and individual event and one that you have only so much control over. However, 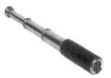 don't lose heart, you can make a big difference in helping to make decisions that will affect the birth – and that is your mission, to do everything within your power to guarantee both the mother and the child are protected and taken care of.

Simply speaking, your involvement must be in providing the best possible environment for the birth, and also in providing the best you have to offer in the pregnancy. Man's role covers three main areas: (a) you are the protector of the birth environment, (b) you are the emotional support, and (c) you are protector of the mother and the coming child. You need to learn about this mission to know what dangers really exist and what can be done to reduce those risks. You need to provide your partner as much emotional support as possible – which may also mean that you support others in providing that support. And, as the child coming is yours, you are the welcoming committee. Trying to make your partner feels safe in having this child is probably the largest part of your whole mission. Succeed in that, and you most likely will have no trouble with the rest. Just think of it as providing a safe place for the flight and landing.

Since you are not a woman and never can truly understand what being one is like, just recognize that women need women in this process of birth. As we have it in us to want to protect others, they have it in them to nurture others. Your form of support is different. You become more of a supportive sentry. You keep the peace and stop others from interfering. Make certain that your partner is taken care of by people who will be nurturing especially if you are unable to muster much of that emotional support.

The Smart Wingman

The basis of our story is that childbirth is akin to flying a sortie. The position you have is the wingman. Your job is to ensure the captain of the mission comes through safely. You are the guard searching the sky for danger and obstacles to the mission.

So what does this mission translate in practical terms? First, let's think a bit about what is happening here. What are the inherent dangers approaching? If you entrust your partner and baby to others are they in good hands? Many men cannot deal with these responsibilities and just hand their family's care over to the medical establishment. You may feel very awkward with the childbirth experience. You may reason, the doctors have been through this countless times so everything will be just fine. But is that smart? Have you done enough research? Do you know enough to make any decisions about this?

Your Mental Concept of Birth?

Your mental picture of birth is important. Are you consciously aware of your thoughts on the subject? What do you think of birth? Since birth starts as an intimate experience, do you think it will suddenly shift to a totally analytical or scientific experience? Did you need to study anatomy and physiology texts before you had intercourse? Do you think of childbirth as a medical problem? Is it a cancer or a broken femur? Are there viruses involved? Or is birth the most natural of human experiences?

Birth today has become what it was never intended to become, a medical emergency. Historically more than ninety-nine percent of human life has been born outside of a sterile room. Yes, there are physical dangers involved, but birth is still a natural bodily function and can be seen as the pinnacle of sexual reproduction. Some think of it as the big bang, orgasmic in power. Many of us realize that after we have children that they are just a mixture of our bodies physically and our personalities emotionally. Actually watching a child grow up and picking out their similarities to you and partner (or family members) is a fun and rewarding activity.

When you envision the coming birth, do you see surgical tents, masked surgeons, and IVs? Do you see steel stirrups, and white sheets and needles? Or do you see birthstools, warm blankets, and home? Might your vision include flowers and hugs? These visions often create the actual scenes to come.

Because agreement with your partner is vital, you need to learn what she thinks birth is about and where she sees you fitting in. If she is scheduling a trip to Ontario and you are flying to Dallas, you may have trouble keeping things together. You need to work together on this.

Write a birth plan. There is a book that is titled "Write It Down, Make It Happen." Well birth isn't that simple, but if you don't write it down, you probably can't make it happen, and if you don't write it down together, you will not know what you are supposed to be doing as this thing unfolds.

What Are The Dangers?

If your mission is to protect your partner and the coming child, will you be willing to not think and to trust strangers with their care? The generations previous went that way. Then look what happened. In thirty years, cesarean sections went from 5% to over 30% in North America -- nearly 50% in many hospitals. Technological birth brought about more emergencies and more surgeries and more complications. The cesarean section rate surged with no improvement in maternal or infant mortality – that means the surgeries do not provide a better chance of safety for the child or mother. Mortality rates for mothers and babies have also not improved since 1982, so perhaps the over medicalization of birth has not improved the safety of childbirth, though many in our culture believe the opposite.

As sexual intimacy is a private personal experience, so is birth. Would you want to have intercourse in a sterile environment, with your woman drugged and a surgeon standing at the door, dressed in blue scrubs with a scalpel in hand (in case anything goes wrong)? That is what has happened to birth in this country. Society has given over to the idea that doctors must deliver babies. Whereas, in other places in the world, women are still birthing their babies in homes, huts, and fields – most often without medical assistance. The four industrialized countries with the least amount of deaths of mothers and children have an interesting statistic: over 70% of births occur without doctors. The United States has one of the worst rates of deaths for mothers and children of industrialized, first world nations. American medicine, which ranks so high in other practices, holds 28th place among the developed countries. They only hold first place for the expense of childbirth.

So you have to know something in order for you to help make good decisions if you want the best for those you are protecting, and you need to know that everyone who you speak to isn't going to have the same perspective as you. Many older women were indoctrinated in the medical technical birth philosophy. You just need to use your own head to choose. Don't let others choose for you. Remember you have a lot at stake here. You have a baby and a mother (who is definitely at her most vulnerable). If you mess this up, not protecting their interests, you may find that after the birth, you have lost more than you could possible ever imagine. Yet, if you fly your mission right, you can come out with the world!

Birth as Big Business

Remember money drives a lot of people to tell you things that aren't necessarily better for you. Just think about formula and the poor substitute it is for a woman's breast milk. Science has shown breast milk is vastly superior, but do you know how much money and energy is poured into making you think that the formula is better. It seems that the hook in our society is always not what is best, but what is most convenient. So the generations before bought the lies that formula was best, and you can be assured that marketing is nothing more than skillful brainwashing. Someone made a fortune off that, and they continue to sell that idea overseas today.

So what is the current lie? That birth is an emergency? That the mother and child are at great risk? That you should schedule a safe c-section? Whatever it is, it will be sold by convenience and fear. Remember nothing is to be feared but fear itself. So when someone is trying to manipulate you to make a major decision based on fear, you know they are selling something false.

Hospitals have a break-even point with birth. After a woman has labored past that point, they start losing money. Generally a woman will have active labor from between 10 to 20 hours. With first time deliveries, where this is the woman's first child, the body has a great deal of changing to do. All those ligaments have to stretch, soften and open up for the birth. This takes a great deal of work. Yet many doctors want the process to be sped up. They introduce drugs to push the process faster. Drugs that are not even FDA approved are used to force things along.

That is true of a drug called Cytotec (generic: myspertone). This drug, which is labeled with a warning "This drug should never be used on pregnant women," causes violent contractions of the uterus that in one doctor's words "turns the cervix to mushie." This has been commonly used to induce a woman to start her labor. This is all to get the babies out faster and more efficiently, but what about safety?

Did you know that hospitals that do not have a healthy maternity ward generally face financial collapse? The maternity ward is the moneymaker. That is the business. Hospitals need to turn out as many babies as possible to stay in the black.

Other's Birth Experiences

All around you are men who are now fathers. Pull some aside and you'll find out that they will have their own personal experiences to share. We find that one of the great things about life in general is that we can learn from reading and hearing about other's experiences. Ask some women about birth, and you might not get them 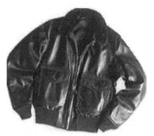 to stop talking about the subject. You could spend the rest of your life learning about other's experiences, and probably the topic is limitless.

We have been through four absolutely different birth experiences. Our oldest daughter was born after major complications, a month's bed rest for Genny, and a cesarean section. The second daughter was born in a hospital with certified nurse midwives. The third was born (water birth) in a free-standing birth center with midwives, and the last was born at home with a midwife. It was these experiences that led us to evaluate and appreciate the diversity of birth experiences. These four scenarios played out in front of us -- observers and participants. We can tell you that each one left a lasting impression on us about how birth is and how it can be handled. You develop some strong feelings after each of these flights.

So learn all you can from the men you come in contact with. Look for the nuggets of wisdom and be free to file their stories away in your mind as you involve yourself in this thing called childbirth.

Flight School

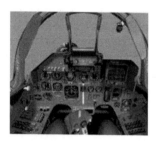 Part of your mission is to learn everything you can about what your role can and should be in the birth. The fact that you are concerned enough to read a book on the subject says a lot of positive things about your character. Remember the easy way out is to do nothing, but with birth at least you have nine months to prepare. Someone once told us that they thought the opposite of love was self love, but then someone else told me that no it was apathy and indecision. So sitting static may be the most damaging thing a person can do. And the reason most people don't act is that they are paralyzed with fear – that old enemy – might as well label it the demon it is.

The brother of apathy must be ignorance. The combination places people in shackles. One cannot act unless they care and if they know what action to take. The ultimate purpose and mission in this thing called childbirth is to provide a safe and protected childbirth environment. If you were not motivated to care about that, then you wouldn't be reading this. The mission of this book is to provide you pertinent information that can help you to fly your mission with commonsense and wisdom. What would the mission be without good intelligence?

Would any of you go down to the car dealer and have the salesmen pick out the car they thought was the best car? That is how childbirth in North America is handled. You go with whatever the insurance will pay for. Everything is geared to the medical establishment's choices. With insurance, many of us don't know we can ask for alternative care or a second opinion. We just expect that everything is sound. It would be totally different if we all had to pay out of our own pocket.

Not many of us shop around when it comes to medical services. Phil had a knee surgery, and he just asked around to find a convenient place. He didn't know the doctor, and can't even recall his name. Insurance paid for everything. We all learn to handle medicine in this way, and that is probably why insurance costs have skyrocketed in the last twenty years.

We are convinced that this invariably corrupts medicine. We are supposed to just trust the system with both our lives and our fortunes. But we all know that there is bad medicine, unethical practices, and poor health care. Don't be hoodwinked into thinking that you don't need to be concerned about a birth as long as it is covered by insurance.

Hospitals are in business to make money. Your insurance covers about anything they do. We remember that we only had to pay a $16 co-pay when Genny ended up having a c-section. That operation and hospital stay cost over $20,000. Remember, the hospitals starts losing money on a birth the longer you are there. They have developed techniques to speed up birth which are both dangerous and cause complications for birthing mothers.

When unnecessary medical interventions are introduced, these tend to have risks which turn into complications. These complications in themselves force more interventions. Take for instance the test for alpha fetoproteins – usually done to see if a baby is mentally retarded. This test is wrong thirty percent of the time. Once the test is run, you have the anxiety of waiting for the results. If the test comes back positive, which means there is a possibility of having a child with Down's syndrome, you then have to make a decision. People can abort the child. They can choose to do an amniocentesis to provide more information – verifying the finding. Amniocentis can cause its own problems – infections, damaging the baby, etc. If you never chose to have the test, accepting whatever baby you've got coming, no anxiety and no danger. But most insurance policies are going to cover these procedures. So what's it to you? Well what if you were told your baby was mentally retarded and aborted it only to learn that they had been wrong. Or what if you had had the amniocentesis done only to damage the baby or kill it – wouldn't you be upset – what do you think your partner would feel. You have to weigh all these decisions out long before you arrive there.

Another favorite intervention technique is to induce labor. This means generally that instead of waiting until labor starts naturally, you force it. Sometimes a woman's body isn't ready to birth yet. But once you chose induction, the woman almost always has to give birth. First, if they broke the bag of waters, then there is a chance that infection can occur. That usually gives you another intervention like pitocin. That means an IV and risk to the baby for fetal distress. Then the next thing you know, they are wheeling your partner to prep for surgery.

Take the epidural as another example. This is a surgical drugging of a woman's lower body. It is a very expensive procedure that requires a doctor called an anesthesiologist. Of course, this is covered by insurance. The process causes complications in about 25% of women. 15 to 35 percent of these women develop fever, which results in diagnostic tests and antibiotic treatment for your baby. 40 percent of women given an epidural have severe backache for hours and days after the birth. 20% have that ache a year later. Yes the drug kills the pain of labor, but what are the consequences of that. 8 to 12% of babies born after their mother is drugged develop hypoxia, which is the deprivation of oxygen to the baby. The stats show women who have had an epidural die 3 times more often than those who don't.

Remember most North American births are handled by surgical doctors. That is their training. Most of them do not attend births until the last minute or unless serious complication begin. They basically order the nurses at the hospital to offer your partner interventions. You as a man better know what risks and complications can result. Protect you partner – remember women have over 5 times greater chance of dying from a cesarean section than any other type of birth, and nearly one in three are having this surgery.

Interventions are covered by your insurance and hospitals will offer you as many as you will take. Usually one intervention attracts another. The hospital makes money from providing medical services. It's like taking your car into a shop and the mechanic says, "Hey, we can do a lube job, rotate your tires and check your fluids; then you find out they have to turn the rotors, your engine needs a ring job and your transmission is leaking.

Birth Machine" is an expression coined by Marsden Wagner, a world renowned neonatologist and epidemiologist who is active in the World Health Organization's Maternal and Child Health division, and is an ardent supporter of midwifery and midwives. The term "Birth Machine," defines the current prominent model of childbirth as a medical model that is characterized by a prevailing use of technology and interventions, often without scientific evidence featuring cesarean sections in a litigious society. The medical model is in direct opposition to the social model of childbirth that is a model recognized by a community involvement in childbirth, an increased use of midwives and a limited use of technology.

The birth machine has you tied down on their timetable. They may make you believe that things are going wrong, when they are just going slowly. They have you thinking that everything is an emergency (why else would you go to the hospital). They tell you they must do such and such procedure (without telling you the inherent risks). Remember that doctor's wants to expedite the birth because they have scheduled full days of appointments. The sooner your partner births the better for them. But labor takes hours and patience (obstetric means to sit and wait).

We know a woman who attended an academic resuscitation class where nurses who work in labor and delivery at hospitals have said that doctors have prescribed upping the dose of pitocin in a mother to cause fetal distress in the child so that they can have a reason for a c-section. This is a fact that cannot be hidden; the nurses are doing everything they can to avoid that type of order, but they are not in charge. The doctors are! These nurses are smart. They articulate between themselves the fact that not all doctors have at heart the best interests of the birthing mother.

You may not feel like challenging your own belief about medicine, but hopefully you will care enough about your coming child and your vulnerable partner to know what true dangers exist in the present day world of birth. Your knowledge about what is happening with birth is essential. The more you understand, the better you are prepared to protect. The care providers you have may be total strangers to you. Should they make your decisions for you? By the time you finish these briefings, you should be able to serve your partner's interests well and make good decisions.

Chapter 3: Knowing the Equipment

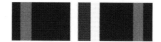

Your Partner's Body

Understanding the female reproductive system can only improve your ability to understand the language of birth and pregnancy. You really don't have to be a genius to take this all in, but without knowing any of this, you may lose the power to be able to protect your child and partner. Believe me you really don't need to have a medical background. You can learn enough to know that when an intervention is introduced how that can impact the process of birth.

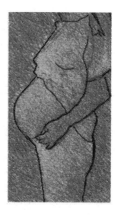

The Uterus

First, do you know what the uterus is? That is the muscular structure that provides the strength to push the baby out of a womb. A ruptured one is not a good thing, and that would require surgery to deal with. However, let's focus on a normal healthy unit. This thing is amazing. It is the strongest muscular structure in any human's body. It has to push a rubbery 6 to 10 pound child through an opening that starts out as tiny as your urethra (place where your pee flows out). The muscles run left and right, up and down. This is the place where all those contractions occur, and the woman really can't control that; at least not like we can flex out biceps and triceps. It is quite incredible to watch one contracting. It looks like Hercules flexing.

One of the most amazing things about childbirth is that this organ increases by about one thousand times to accommodate the growing child. Of course this affects all the standard organs of a woman's body since they all get cramped up. Many of the discomforts of pregnancy are due to this growth. Have patience with your partner. Her bladder especially gets a raw deal. She may also find it difficult to breathe, and she may have heartburn. The whole thing just accelerates near the end of the pregnancy until you will constantly hear, "I want this baby out!" Can you imagine the affect of carrying an 8 to 9 pound ball around plus a 2 to 3 pound placenta certainly would be uncomfortable for you.

The Cervix

The cervix is another vital part of the woman's birth equipment. This is a donut-like end of the womb (or uterus). It is the pathway through which the sperm must pass. After conception, it is still the exit site for the birth. So this very narrow opening must stretch wide enough and become thin enough to release the baby into vagina and then out. The cervix sits at the bottom of the birth canal. When the baby's head is engaged in the canal, this begins pressuring the cervix open. This process takes some women quit a long time, but, for others, they have it happen rapidly. You can't tell. So know your cervix. When it is 5 centimeters open, that's half way, and most consultants will tell you that now the labor is serious.

The Mucous Plug

This is a growth of capillaries and mucous that is found plugging the hole in the cervix, stopping all foreign matter from entering the uterus. It is created after conception and falls out at the end of pregnancy when the cervix starts preparing for birth.

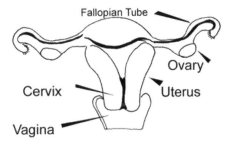

The Perineum

The perineum, a small tissue running between the anus and the labia, is not without place in the process of birth because it too has to stretch to let the baby out; therefore you should know enough about this to be aware of what the medical world thinks about that. Currently there is a simple operation, called an episiotomy, where doctors slice the end of the vagina to open the space for the baby to come through. In women who have no episiotomy, sometimes the vagina will not flex enough and the tissue will tear, but with a cut, often tearing just follows the incision, producing an even nastier tear. Midwives often spend the time and effort applying warm compresses and massaging warm oil into the perineum to improve is elasticity and help stretch the tissue.

The Vagina

The vagina is the part of the reproductive system that is mostly a cavern. The cervix sits at the back and is the door to and from the uterus. The vagina is another area that can tear during the birth process especially if the child does something unusual like stick out an arm up over its head, thereby forcing more than the designed need for stretching. When things don't stretch, they tear. This doesn't happen a lot, but at least you know something about what could happen. The tears are most always on the outer edges of the labia.

The Vulva

The vulva is the external portion of the woman's reproductive system. It includes the labia, major and minor, and the clitoris.

The Placenta

The placenta is an organ that is created only during a pregnancy. This is like a special life support system that sits inside the womb passing nutriments from the mother's blood supply into the baby and removing waste products from the baby's blood supply and dumping them into the mother's blood. A healthy placenta is significant to growing a healthy baby. The umbilical cord from the baby attaches to this. The baby is born first, and then the placenta is the main piece of the after birth. It detaches from the inside of the uterus and comes out. The way it detaches is highly important. A good detach and the whole thing comes out with little complication, but if it refuses to release, then there is serious trouble.

The Umbilical Cord

The umbilical cord is a series of three vessels that run between the baby's abdomen and the placenta. The cute little belly button on all of us is formed when the cord is snipped and tied. We suspect that Adam and Eve didn't have one, but everyone else gets one. This cord of life can be a real problem during the birthing process since the cord can tangle around the baby or become compressed during contraction somehow cutting of air supply. Just think of it like a cord on your vacuum. If it gets wrapped around a neck, not only can it inhibit a normal birth, but also it can cause fetal distress. When the cord gets pinched, then the flow of oxygen is compromised.

The Business of Hormones

The complexity of how the human body works is wrapped up in a variety of chemical exchanges and processes. Pregnancy and childbirth are all about hormones. Hormones are powerful and change the way your partner feels, acts and grows. You may have heard of estrogen and progesterone. Pregnancy multiplies these hormones. Progesterone increases by more that 250 times its original levels. Estrogen goes up 20 to 30 times. These chemicals radically shift after birth, especially after the milk comes into your partner's breasts. This shift in chemicals can produce emotional volatility and open the door for post partum depression.

Hormones are what bring about birth and what can stop birth from progressing. Oxytocin is the main ingredient. The non-thinking part of the brain, in conjunction with the endocrine system, sets off a long series of involved chemical processes – but those processes all have an enemy, called adrenaline that will put the brakes on and curb a labor.

Additional Physiological Changes

As your partner's body is changing, many physiological alterations occur. The volume of blood moves to 14 pints, or 45% higher than pre-pregnancy. This change means there has to be enough red blood cells, so iron is important in the diet. As the blood volume increases, there also has to be a proportional increase in sodium intake to help retain those fluids.

As this amount of blood has to be oxygenated and pumped throughout the body, the lungs and heart have a greater workload. Your partner's pulse rate will increase 10 to 15 beats per minute. Exercise just improves the amount of deep breathing and adds to the quality of oxygen in her system. Walks are great for bonding and for improving your partner's circulation and air intake.

Another change is that the kidneys are filtering a great amount of blood as well, and since the wastes from the child are now part of the materials being filtered, so the workload of these organs hits overdrive. This also connects to the bladder's overload. Pregnant women live half their lives in the bathroom.

The important thing to know about those kidneys is that they also eliminate the good with the bad as they take on this greater load. These renal functions drop glucose (energy), important minerals, vitamins and folic acid. Thus, universally, women need better diets, vitamin intake, etc. This is where you come in. You can't carry part of this physiological need, but you can help your partner to eat healthy foods.

Ligaments hold everything together in the back, pelvis and the hips of your partner, but, when she is pregnant, these joints will change due to hormonal changes. These changes are in anticipation of the coming labor when they will need to mold to provide smooth passage through. By the 16th week, the pelvic brim can be tipped by the force of the baby against it. This can cause a great deal of strain, so proper posture is needed to lessen the strain. There are exercises designed with this in mind such as squats. In childbirth the muscles of the inner thighs are paramount in importance. A woman's pelvis significantly expands for baby's exit in the squatting position. Encourage her to incorporate squatting as an exercise and to utilize squatting in her daily activities, especially when picking thing up. Stronger thighs mean easier births. She should be building her stamina up with consistent exercise so that she will be strong for the birth. You will find that as the pregnancy rolls along, your partner will become more and more uncomfortable, so initiating exercise from the start will help reduce some of the strains of a pregnancy. However, with all that said, exercise in pregnancy should never be jarring to the body and the uterus as that can cause miscarriage.

Other changes affect your partner's skin hair and nails. The most noticeable and common are the discoloration of the skin, especially in areas such as the areolas and genital region. Sometimes these changes will never revert back. Oftentimes there is a skin darkening that appears as a half inch line from the pubic bone straight up to the chest – this usually just fades away. Most of these pigmentation changes disappear, so don't worry about it, and encourage your partner not to worry. Other undetermined changes in the oiliness of the skin can cause pimples, so that too is another cosmetic change, which may require your understanding. The word here is care -- to build up your partner and ignore these insignificant physical changes which may be huge to her.

A cosmetic change which may be more permanent is stretch marks. The increase in certain hormones causes your partner's skin to change. Basically the structure of the skin is made up of collagen strands. These bundles are undermined by fat accumulations especially around the hips, bust and abdomen. These markings may be a pinkish color during pregnancy and silvery afterwards. They may never go away, so your partner's perfect complexion may take a step down, and this could really upset her. It does not happen to every woman, but it happens often so reassure your partner that it is just part of the life cycle. Some of us become prematurely bald, grey, and wrinkled. Stretch marks are just part of the aging process. That is the mature and responsible way of thinking of it, but don't expect your partner to not be upset by these changes to her appearance. Think of them as badges of courage or honor.

Additional changes may affect your partner's hair. Some women's straight hair turns curly, and this may stay that way after the birth. While some women find their hair getting healthier looking, others find their hair becomes lifeless and greasy. In the later days of a pregnancy certain glands produce more oil in the scalp. Whatever the case, the big change may come after the birth and up to 18 months later, as you may find your partner's hair thinning. This is because the hair is normally on course to be replaced at let's say 90 percent growing, 10 percent falling out. Then during the pregnancy the hair just all grows – hair, that should have be dying, stays healthy. Yet, when the hormones shift back, hair loss resumes. This may become alarming for your partner, but never let her fear because it's normal and no woman goes bald due to a pregnancy.

The Signals of Birth

Know one really understands what the real sign is for the coming birth. People talk about water breaking, and contractions starting. But even these can be false signs. There are contractions all through the pregnancy though your partner may not feel them; they are termed Braxton Hicks and occur every 20 minutes throughout the pregnancy. During the last month, they can be thought to be quite strong and can be thought to be the real thing – this is called false labor. Of course, if that occurs, you have to know something about infections and temperatures.

So how does a woman know when it is time? That is a good thing to go over. The best clue that a woman is in active labor is that the cervix is thinning and opening, and not just a little bit, but more like half way. Some women go rapidly, and the power of the contractions and the fact that the woman can't talk through those contractions is a telltale sign.

But again, the usual course is that leading up to the time when things really get cooking, there will be some contractions – it's like preliminary exercises. Water breaking – like there's a flood, that's another clue, but not until there are consistent contractions do you really know. Even then these may peter out within a couple hours.

A woman, who has already had one child rapidly, may need to be closely watched near the end of the gestational time period since she might go quickly again. But, that isn't necessarily so. One thing that is for sure is that if you've scheduled a cesarean section, then that's what time the baby will come.

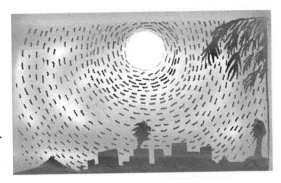

You'll hear all sorts of tales about what starts this. You'll hear full moons or certain weather patterns or eating certain foods. But research isn't conclusive. It appears that it might just be the child who says, "Hey, I want better food than I get in here. Give me something good to eat!" The only sure way to know it was true labor is after that baby is born.

Equipment Processes

But let's get back on track here. The natural childbirth requires some physiological changes to take place before the child can be born. The fact remains that the baby has to come through a birth canal via a cervix. The baby has to get lined up in this canal first. It's like locking in the space shuttle to the orbiting space station. They say the baby has dropped, and that means things are lining up for the landing. This is usually pretty obvious to all involved. Your partner may waddle around. Just try walking holding a softball between your legs.

Then that old cervix has to loosen up, and that requires both physiological and chemical changes. Early on labor will jamb the baby's head against the cervix, pressing and pressing against it. Then the hormones that are being released will begin to soften the cervix. We really don't think anyone is doing any scientific studies during actual births as to the chemical changing of this tissue. So it is just possible that tampering with this process is just that: tampering.

Doctors and midwives have a chemical called pitocin (a synthetic oxytocin) usually administered intravenously (IV) to bolster and strengthen the contractions. They usually administer that when labor isn't progressing. A way to naturally increase human oxytocin in the blood is through stimulating a woman's nipples or stimulating the roof of her mouth (French kissing or sucking the thumb). Oxytocin is the "love" hormone, and that is what the pitocin is emulating. Some people feel that the way the baby got inside is the way you get it out, but remember that is when labor isn't progressing, and there are a myriad of reasons for that. Regardless the medical establishment will try to put birth on their timetable and that is what pit is about. For women to birth they need to be relaxed and secure. Sexually women are more apt to be turned on when they feel cherished and cared for. Coming home after work for sex with the woman might be the man's idea of heaven, but women aren't turned on like a light switch. They need the flowers, the soothing romantic music, the gentleness and the wining and dining before they warm up to intimate relations. Birth is like that. Women need the right mood, the right place and the right person around before they feel free to birth.

Now you understand that you can see there is a conflict in how labor is pushed versus encouraged. The door to the womb, which is thick and tight, has to be pressed thin and open for the baby's head to get through. The uterus's job isn't to beat upon this baby, but to slowly and surely eject the baby out. The baby helps as well, as two reflexes come into play. One is that when the feet are touched, the baby straightens out its legs. The other is that when the baby's head is compressed, it wiggles its neck.

Now before the baby gets engaged in top of the birth canal, there is some important positioning that occurs. First, the baby has to be turned head down. But the way the baby faces is also important. You want that lined up. Professionals should be able to tell you and your partner where things sit. This is important to ensure the birth process can go most smoothly. Get a baby breech and a talented pro can sometimes get things turned around, given enough time. Get a baby on the back (set up for back labor, a very painful situation which weakens a woman) and you've got trouble from the start. A pro can help adjust things before a birth. Make sure your professional can handle these things. If you ask the right questions and get solid answers back, you will be able to gage the skill of your professional.

This is a simple version of how it all works. You just need to do all you can before the labor and delivery to improve the chance of a successful natural childbirth. Knowing the equipment helps to ward off anxiety. Also knowing that you have engaged well trained assistance can further create a sense of security and confidence. A good pilot knows his options.

The Progress of Labor

For many reasons, many women start laboring, then stop, then start again. The smooth progression of labor doesn't always happen. Many care providers handle this issue differently. The concern is over the failure to progress (FTP) occurs in the second stage of labor. Now there may be many reasons for FTP, but two major reasons exist. The first is fear! See women aren't machines; they are people, and people are bodies, souls and spirits. Birth is a physiological dimension, yet higher dimensions affect things. Fear actually causes negative physiological conditions.

Now let's look at the uterus and understand the basic physiology of what is does during birth. First of all three sets of muscle groups exist. Two are stimulated from oxytocin. This chemical stimulates the contractions. The diagonal or oblique group points down to the bottom of the uterus at the cervix. These muscles have one main part – they open the cervix up for the passage of the baby. At the same time the oxytocin is stimulating another set of muscles, which sit like latitude (up and down) lines on the globe. When they contract they push down and move the baby out. The two sets work together to efface and dilate the cervix.

Yet, there at the meridian is a third set of uterine muscles that don't promote labor progress. These muscles do not run off oxytocin. Now what is the design of a set of labor muscles that will pull against the other two groups? They are designed to stop labor. But why? Fear. These muscles respond to adrenaline. Just imagine your partner giving birth in the woods. Then a bear arrives. The muscles stop the labor and she can get up and run. However, the fact that your partner isn't living in the pristine 13th century America, shows that something else is causing fear than a wild animal.

The whole risk management scheme that is predominant in American childbirth is saturated with fear. Hearing a woman in transition in a hospital is sometimes enough to shut down birth, or maybe it was a screeching defective wheel on a gurney. There are a myriad of things going on in the hospital that bring fear. For other women, not being in the hospital is going to cause them to feel afraid. These attitudes can cause problems. First of all, by subjecting themselves to the idea that a home birth is the only way, resistance is built for transfer when serious complications arise. As reported, 4.4 percent of births at freestanding birth centers with midwives result in surgical intervention, and none of these are high-risk births in the first place. Then, as commonly documented, many women end up with a cesarean in the hospital that statistically shouldn't have trouble. Fear abounds when understanding is insufficient.

Whatever you do, you must position yourself to help eliminate fear. Fear can really screw up a birth. The environment of birth should be safe for women. They should feel comfortable so they can focus of letting go and letting the birth happen. Even when a woman is a ready to birth, these physiological factors can shut it down. Genny told Phil, once when she was laboring with her first VBAC (vaginal birth after cesarean), that she had to get herself into a place (the shower) where she could de-stress and get into the birth.

Remember fear can come from actual physical stimulus, or through psychological issues. Women who were abused, raped, or molested can bind up with internal fears they can't even reason through during labor. Other situations shut it down too: loud or screeching noises, people who bring terrible news or undesired news, or a change that is unexpected, like a shift of staff, can trigger the brakes. Women talk about hearing other women laboring in other labor suites upsetting them. All of these factors can be mitigated in planning well, though not all can be foreseen. Many men describe birth as an unexpected ride. The whole point here is to consider doing all you can do to eliminate the dangers as best you can.

Now another major reason for failure to progress is that the cervix is not prepared for the birth. Physiologically the uterus may be turned up and on with either natural or injectable oxytocin. But, if the cervix is hard and tight, so that it can't loosen up, you will find that no matter how much a woman's uterus does that it will fail to get the doors open for labor.

Naturally, women don't normally go into full labor when their cervix is not ready. Women who have not had babies, can easily mistake their bodies signals. They can be thinking that this is it, and run off to the hospital. Midwives are often called out to homes to check on women who think "this is it," only to have to turn around and go home – sometimes nothing more happens for a couple of weeks. So we men really are placed in an awkward situation. With our third birth we lived 65 miles away from the birth center (the only facility where we could have a VBAC). At 4 in the morning Genny told Phil that she was ready and that he should get the car started. Phil called the care giver who responded that he would know when it was the right time when Genny couldn't talk during a contraction. Phil went back to sleep. When he got downstairs at 8 am to make something to eat for breakfast, Genny was in the kitchen. He asked her how she was doing. She couldn't say anything as she was having a good strong contraction. But as soon as she finished, she threw a full loaf of bread across the room at him. Then he knew it was time to load the car and go.

Phil has seen Genny begin and stop, begin and stop, then have several days pass before the real thing engaged. Genny has seen many other women experience the same thing. A good test between real labor and false labor is having her get into a tub of warm water. If the contractions come to a standstill then you know it was a practice exercise, and she can go back to her normal daily routine.

If you fail to progress in the hospital after you arrive prematurely, don't think you can't go home. They may not inform you of this, but you can go home and return when you are in more active labor. If your partner's cervix is less than 5 centimeters dilated, then go home, especially if things have stopped progressing.

The only ways we know of helping to soften up the cervix safely is to provide certain internal nutrients or external chemicals. As you may have heard, by doing what got the baby in there in the first place may be the only thing you as a man can do to help get the baby out. As mentioned, breast stimulation releases oxytocin, the chemical for turning on the uterus for contractions. Your semen is also supposedly helpful in softening up the cervix. Making love to a very pregnant partner can help to bring about the onset of labor, but we aren't making any promises. However being tender helps her psychologically and as mentioned certain natural chemicals may help prepare her for the time of labor. Remember the romance a woman likes can help her mind to relax for the release of the love hormone. Wining and dining, flowers and caresses may be all she needs to help her start. According to research done on sexual orgasm, both males and females get a big surge of oxytocin before they climax, and the same is true in delivering vaginally.

For someone to be comfortable to have an orgasm in front of other people, that person has to be focused and very comfortable with the people there. These psychological issues seem to be overlooked. No, it isn't the same, but in many ways it still is. First your partner wants to be with those she is at ease with. That is why working with a person through the whole birth is helpful. That level of care helps a woman feel comfortable when vulnerable and that improves the ability to birth naturally.

Chapter 4: Testing, Testing, 1, 2, 3

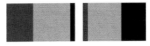

You should know about tests that are used today. They were developed by the medical community to provide you and your partner important information. Your medical professionals use these tests to help determine many things like the health of the mother and baby.

Confirmation

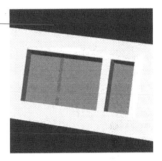

Pregnancy tests, obviously, are used. Some women buy one any time they are late for starting menstruation. Men never have that anxiety. One of the main stays of the women's liberation movement and the pro choice power is that women want control over their ability to decide when they will get pregnant. This is a big deal, so treat the pregnancy test quietly. You may, at first, not care whether or not she is pregnant, but she will. Respect that!

The basic signs to tell when a woman is pregnant are simple: missed periods, frequent urination, morning sickness, changes in the breasts, etc; however, the first test your partner may get is one sold at your local pharmacy – the cost is nominal. These home kits take a sample of urine and check it for a chemical (human chorionic gonadotrophin), if the tests presents positive, usually the stick has a blue color. If you wait two weeks after the first days of a missed menstruation cycle, this improves the chances of the test proving accurate. The urine test, arranged with a healthcare professional, involves sending a sample of your partner's morning urine to the lab. Negative results for either a home kit or a lab test do not necessarily mean you do not have a pregnancy either. After the eight week of a missed period, your healthcare provider may perform an internal examination that can conclusively determine if there is a pregnancy. Also a blood test exists that is very accurate and can be ordered up if need be.

You may find out immediately from your partner that she is pregnant. She is the one most likely to know if her body has changed. Yet the tests help to take the anxiety of the whole thing away.

Remember that this issue of controlling when one is pregnant is a huge deal to women, and one that we guys may never appreciate. Once your partner knows she has become pregnant, you may see a variety of emotional reactions. You may see bitterness, anger, depression or joy and excitement – or all of them depending on what she is thinking about. So that is why you need to handle this test with kid gloves.

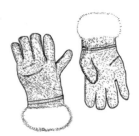

More Urine Tests

Every time your partner goes in for a monthly prenatal visit, she may be asked to provide a sample of her urine. This test is used to determine if your partner is passing protein, sugar or ketones. Protein may be a sign of pre-eclampsia. Sugar or ketones may indicate diabetes. If there are problems with the kidneys, these tests may also give forewarning. Ketones are passed when a woman is not eating properly as well. Her body begins sort of digesting itself. With morning sickness, this can be common since she may not be able to eat anything.

Blood Tests

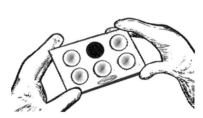

Besides telling what blood group (in case of emergency) your partner is in these tests, they usually are run to determine RH blood group, check hemoglobin levels, detect German measles antibodies, detect syphilis, sickle cell disease and thalassemia.

RH compatibility is important. If the baby is positive and the mother negative RH, then a negative RH body will fight the positive as a foreign cells which migrate from the baby. The negative RH mother will produce antibodies to defend herself and can damage the baby – this usually doesn't happen until after the first childbirth; however, your partner should be checked especially if she is negative RH – this occurs in 20% of the population.

Pregnancy demands hemoglobin. With more blood circulating in your partner's body, her hemoglobin can drop below 10gm. Your place is to help encourage her to eat iron rich foods and to take her supplemental iron and folic acid.

If your partner's blood test shows raised levels of alpha fetoproteins between week 16 and 18, when normally they should be low, then this may lead to evidence of neural tube defect. If they are usually the amniotic fluid is tested through amniocentesis (see below). The alpha fetoproteins at this time period could mean there are two babies or that there may be a defect such as spina bifida or abnormal brain development.

Another test now routinely handled is for the presence of strep in the vagina after the 36th week of pregnancy. If the test returns positive for the strep, then your health care provider may want to run an IV of antibiotics during the labor, to fight off any infection. Some think that by keeping the vagina clean that this precaution is unnecessary, so it depends on your health care practitioner's point of view. Remember you and your partner make those choices!

Blood Pressure

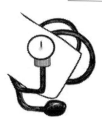

Abnormal blood pressure can become a real issue in pregnancy. Normal is around 120 over 80. If there is an issue of hypertension or high blood pressure, this can indicate problems like pre-eclampsia. Bed rest is advised if it cannot be kept down. Any abnormal diastolic figure will be a concern for your partner's health care provider.

More Extensive Tests

Many tests done during pregnancy predict the health of your coming child. Genetic problems are serious. Taking care of a mentally retarded child, a child with Down's and other genetic problems is a tough road to hoe. Many people, out of religious conviction, will avoid all these types of tests, saying they don't care. Others will abort any child they think is genetically problematic. It is a not easy to decide, but make sure your decision is the best one for you. Today, more women are waiting to have their children, and, the later they wait, the more chance of genetic problems.

Alpha-Fetoprotein

Alpha-Fetoprotein (AFP) is a protein produced by the fetal liver and yolk sac. It is present in the maternal blood system (MSAFP) and also in the amniotic fluid (amniotic fluid AFP). Amniotic fluid AFP is gathered from an amniocentesis. The studies of AFP levels demonstrate numerous things however what AFP studies demonstrate well is the presence of fetal body wall defects such as neural tube defects as in spina bifida. When the neural tube is open, it allows AFP to exit the fetus, or leak from the open wall and circulate in larger amounts in the amniotic fluid.

Obstetric Ultrasound

Ultrasound is used in determining the age of the baby, the position of the placenta and in determining the date of delivery. Many people like to learn if they are going to have a boy or a girl. This technology sends sound waves into a body and gives a fairly accurate picture of the baby in utero. You may accompany your partner to this appointment, so you too can ask questions about what you are seeing. Most technicians are happy to point out the organs of the developing baby – later dates will make all of this easier to see and understand.

Ultrasound equipment is used though it has never been proven safe (efficacy), nor has it been proven effective. This routine work is done at the approximate cost of $70-$80 million per year, about $300 per scan as presented by Dr. Sarah Buckley in her literature on ultrasound in Mothering Magazine September 2000. Though medical literature states that Doppler ultrasound is excellent at measuring fetal heart pulsation and blood flow, "evidence does not, at the present time, support the use of Doppler ultrasound in clinical obstetric practice" (Neilson & Grant 1991, p.430). Other scientific reviews recommend only using ultrasound technology in high-risk populations. And presently no evidence exists that supports routine prenatal ultrasound screens, despite a 1999 Senate Committee report from Australia "Rocking the Cradle" that recommended the cost benefit of routine prenatal ultrasound be assessed.

For a condition called intrauterine growth retardation (IUGR) clinicians still routinely screen by using ultrasound, though studies have shown that repeated measurement of fundal height by midwives is more accurate. Besides 80% of the tests for these conditions turn out incorrect as it is. Therefore the level of anxiety and fear that this causes women is ignored though it has been shown that stress and anxiety have a negative effect on the pregnancy. Furthermore a link has been uncovered that demonstrates a connection with frequent prenatal ultrasound and IUGR. One Australian study reported in the British Journal of Obstetrics Gynecology found that women who undergo 5 or more ultrasound are 30% more likely to develop IUGR, than women who do not.

> Although ultrasound is expensive, routine scanning is of doubtful efficacy and the procedure has not been proven safe, this technology is widely used and its use is increasing rapidly, without control. Nevertheless, health policy is slow to develop. No country is known to have developed policies with regard to standards neither for machines nor for training and certification of the operators. A few industrialized countries have begun to respond to the data showing lack of efficacy for routine scanning of all pregnant women. (Marsden Wagner, p. 89)

A study done in 1993 went on to prove that there was no efficacy to routine scanning during pregnancy. In other words, the regular use of ultrasound equipment does nothing to improve the outcome of birth. Yet since it is part of a billion dollar industry, which is covered by every insurance policy, and since it replaces a more traditional approach of taking measurements by hand, doctors rely on this technology.

Besides using ultrasound to randomly screen for odd developments, doctors use the equipment for screening the developing baby for fetal heart monitoring and fetal movement monitoring; but neither has been shown to give accurate results.

The concern with ultrasound

We know of two ways that ultrasound waves affect tissue, from a 1998 report from the American Institute of Ultrasound Medicine Bioeffects. First the ultrasound beam emitted by the transducer (that is the part of the ultrasound equipment that is placed next to the skin) actually raises the temperature of the area that is highlighted by about 1 degree Celsius. The second area of concern is what is known as cavitation. Cavitation is where the normal pouches of gas exist in living tissue are pulsed to the point that they collapse. When this happens, as in the process of an ultrasound, extremely high degrees of temperature in the pockets of gas create potentially toxic chemical products. Through many position papers over the years the International Childbirth Education Association, ICEA, has stated that ultrasound most likely has an affect on neurological and behavioral development. ACOG in their practice guidelines recommends routine prenatal ultrasound for low risk women are to be reserved only for incidences where there is a specific medical indication for the ultrasound.

Doppler Fetoscope Devices

Many Health Care practitioners utilize a hand-held Doppler fetoscope device to listen to the baby's heart beat. These fetoscopes are appliances that operate on ultrasound as well. These devices transmit the equivalent of 35 minutes worth of real-time ultrasound in only one minute of Doppler exposure according to "Understanding Lab Work in the Childbearing Year." Some concerns exist about the degree of this exposure on the developing infant. The same material can be gathered from a real-time ultrasound screen with less exposure than the fetoscope Doppler and at later dates in the pregnancy from a fetoscope, a special stethoscope designed for listening to the baby's heart beat through the mother's abdomen.

So before you have an ultrasound or consent to prenatal use of a Doppler fetoscope, consider why these are being recommended to you or why you might request this use of ultrasound and determine the risk-to-benefit value for your family. Are the benefits of the results in the accuracy of the interpretation of an ultrasound and the exposure of an ultrasound upon your unborn child worth the risk of receiving the scan, or the Doppler exposure? No tests have proven that this scanning is healthy for the baby, and none of the tests it is used for are accurate. Countless couples are given misinformation regarding their unborn child based on inaccurate readings or inconclusive scans. This decision like so many others with regard to prenatal testing must be answered with the question of what you would do with its results. So choose wisely.

Fetoscopy

Fetoscopy is performed by inserting an endoscope, a tiny telescope, through the abdominal wall and into the uterus. A health care practitioner then can have direct visualization of the fetus and is able to observe malformations such as spina bifida and cleft palate (not properly formed mouth/lip). Fetal blood samples can be obtained to determine the presence of blood disorders. Also fetal skin biopsies can be taken to identify skin disorders. Fetoscopy is usually not done until the fifteenth week and when there are serious concerns brought up. The more technological oriented your environment, the higher chance that this type of technology will be employed. Fetoscopy provides the means for highly advanced perinatal care for the unborn child, offering clinicians the vehicle to administer antibiotics to a fetus exposed to toxoplasmosis or to perform surgery to repair spina bifida if the repair can be made to the fetus.

Screening for Chromosomal Abnormality

These tests are usually run frequently when a woman is at risk of having a child with a life threatening or life altering genetic defect. Such instances are women who are 35 and older, women who have had several miscarriages, women who have had previous pregnancies affected by chromosomal defects and lastly women who have genetic defects themselves. The fact is that for women who are older the likelihood of having a child with chromosomal abnormalities astronomically increases. Serious consideration by you and your partner needs to occur before you consent to these tests. The two of you will need to contemplate what the relevance of the tests results mean and what you would do with these results, if anything while keeping in mind that screening tests do not diagnose anything. Their results are indicative of whether or not further, more invasive testing is warranted. One needs to bear in mind that some invasive tests carry their own risk of miscarriage also.

Triple Screen

A multiple marker screening or triple screen is a screening for open neural tube defects, and chromosomal disorders such as Down's syndrome and trisomy 18 or Edwards's syndrome. The triple screen gets its name from the three studies that are done from a sample of maternal blood AFP, HCG, and Estriol. Estriol E3 is the chief estrogen in a pregnant woman produced by the mother the fetus and placenta. The results of these three studies are considered along with the factors of maternal age, weight, race, and gestation of pregnancy to produce a figure representing a probability of chromosomal disorders.

The timing for the triple screen is at 15 to 20 weeks of gestation. The optimum time for the test rendering the best results in accuracy is at 16-18 weeks of gestation. This test is an option for all parents to consider. It becomes especially significant for parents to contemplate if any of following issues exist (1) a family history of birth defects, (2) advanced maternal age, (3) the use of drugs detrimental to the unborn baby by a mother while unknowingly pregnant, (4) for a mother with insulin dependant diabetes, (5) a viral infection during the course of pregnancy, or (6) maternal exposure to significant radiation levels.

Amniocentesis

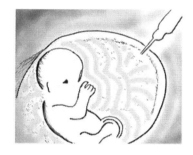

The amniotic fluid contains cells from the baby that give good clues as to the baby's condition. Amniocentesis can detect spina bifida, mongolism or Down's syndrome and is a routine test for women over 35. It is also a test that can detect other abnormalities such as RH incompatibility. These tests are also run if there is a history of abnormalities. Around 75 genetic disorders can be tested – through chromosome analysis. The test is done after 16 weeks gestation. Amniocentesis is excellent for assessing the maturity of a fetus evaluating in particular the maturity of the fetus's lungs. This is an issue of great importance when prematurely is threatened and a decision needs to be made whether or not to allow the pregnancy to continue or to go ahead with an early delivery. The test is performed by advancing a needle through the mother's abdominal and uterine walls to the amniotic fluid under the guidance of an ultrasound image. With the needle in place amniotic fluid is withdrawn for study. The procedure has a minimum miscarriage rate, but it is intrusive. Researchers at the University of California, San Francisco found a miscarriage rate after amniocentesis of 0.83%. Waiting for the results may be the hardest part of the whole affair. This is where your constant assurance is needed. This is a serious test, and that can weigh on anyone's mind.

CVS

Chorionic Villus Sampling CVS is a test used to diagnose chromosomal abnormalities within the first trimester. The test may be performed earlier than amniocentesis. Chronic villi are present from 8 to 12 weeks of gestation. The intricacy of the CVS demands extensive experience to be performed safely. If this is a procedure that you and your partner are interested in because of the earlier timing that this test provides, make certain that you and your physician are comfortable with the confidence level of the physician in performing this test. The alternative is to wait a few more weeks for an amniocentesis to be performed at 16 weeks. The extensive procedure of CVS is performed under the guidance of an ultrasound where a special collection tube called a cannula is inserted through the vagina into the cervix and uterus. The cannula is maneuvered in to place at the site of the developing placenta where 3 or more villous samples are withdrawn for sampling. These samples of the chronic villi, the preliminary construction of the placenta, are understood to reflect chromosomes from the fetus enzymes and DNA. If the ultrasound demonstrates that the chronic villi is difficult to access from the cervix, then the samples may be obtained through the abdomen in much the same way an amniocentesis is performed. Studies have shown that after CVS, a higher likelihood to have increased levels of AFP exists. The same study out of University of California, San Francisco that provided the data of miscarriage rates after an amniocentesis of 0.83% recorded a miscarriage rate for women following CVS to be 3.12%

(See table on next page).

Table: Chromosomal Deviations

Age	Chance in 1000 For Down's Syndrome	Chance in 1000 For All Chromosomal Abnormality
21	1 in 1520	
23	1 in 1450	
25	1 in 1350	
27	1 in 1200	
29	1 in 1010	
30	1 in 890	
31	1 in 775	
32	1 in 660	
33	1 in 545	
34	1 in 445	
35	1 in 355	1 in 115
36	1 in 300	1 in 85
37	1 in 220	1 in 65
38	1 in 165	1 in 50
39	1 in 125	1 in 39
40	1 in 90	1 in 30
41	1 in 70	1 in 22
42	1 in 50	1 in 17
43	1 in 40	1 in 13

Chapter 5: Understanding the Captain

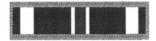

Birth is a pinnacle of life for most women, and, therefore, it should be significant to men. The heightened awareness of life and the added stress and joy the event can bring clearly change the dynamics of your relationship. As you enter into the time of pregnancy and the coming birth, you may learn a great deal about your partner. Understanding her is a key to making sure you are providing her with your best.

Communications Center

First and foremost you need to think that most women are emotional people. Women are more in touch with their feelings and their intuition. We men are kind of numb or dumb. We feel, but we are not moved to tears easily or readily. Now if you've been around women during their menstrual cycle, you know that the level of emotion increases tenfold during that 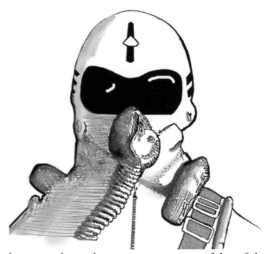 time of the month. Pregnancy changes these hormones measurably. It's like nine month's discharge of emotional energy. The last hours of the labor are a time of profound release, so you can imagine the affect of completing the birth.

You know that being sensitive to your partner during her time of the month is a very wonderful thing for her and improves your relationship. Say the wrong thing, and you'll have an exponential increase in your own turmoil. By saying the wrong thing in the pregnancy you will get turmoil to the "nth" power. The postpartum adjustment also requires diligence and extra sensitive care as your partner's hormones return to the pre-pregnancy levels. Genny likens the hormonal fluctuations after delivery to Chicago O'Hare airport flights as so many hormones are dropping off and so many hormones are coming up.

Since your mission has been established, you choose whether you want to be a highly supportive man. If you want the best, you will learn to screen out all thoughts and all messages of negativity, sarcasm, criticism, and hold yourself in control. Wisdom writes, "The perfect man is the one who has control of his tongue."

If you feel that you have thoughts of biting criticism or other harmful ideas, you may be experiencing your own negative thoughts and feelings. You may find that under all of this that you are vulnerable, afraid and not prepared for the up-and-coming birth. Many times our internal systems that help us control our emotions are not something we are aware of. We may be masters of our feelings. By force of will we hold our feelings down or tune them out. Despite our tough armor, big events like birth, death, disaster, loss of job, etc. can turn our strong shell into a gelatinous form of quivering nerves. Birth and pregnancy may bring out some of the best emotions of life or unfortunately the worst. We may be men, but strong emotions can flatten us like an explosion.

So, since your mission is to protect the mother and child, you need to make it your resolve to ensure that all emotions expressed are healthy and nurturing to help maintain the environment of love, respect and adoration you have for birth and for the relationships you are establishing with the mother and child.

So what do you do if you feel rotten and angry and frustrated?

Since emotions are usually fleeting in us, you might just capture them down in a journal. Phil finds that when he places his intimate thoughts into a journal, that the act itself helps him to come to resolve the problems plaguing him. Having a confidant in your life is another way of dealing with the same. You may need a person who you trust impeccably with your deepest, darkest and intimate secrets. Being able to say everything that comes out of that scary place of your emotional black hole is a very therapeutic and healing. You could even contact a family counselor who has dealt with men's issues especially for dealing with the coming birth. Good counselors are able to draw out the venom of the soul and help focus your desires to rid yourself of all negative emotional baggage and hurt. You may be surprised to see that your fears of the coming birth are actually expressions of a deeper hurt in your own life.

So get counseling, share your soul, and write out your emotions before they interfere with your loving relationship with the mother to be.

Friendly Fire

Your partner is an individual who has her own background with all its associated emotions, thoughts and perceptions. Pregnancy and childbirth are experiences that heighten a woman's vulnerability, which sometimes leads to the release of anxieties, fears and frustrations. In other words, the captain may let loose and no matter how close you are, you should be prepared for a messy time. Just as the woman's body must release physical wastes before the birth, you should expect some negative releases during pregnancy and during the childbirth.

What is essential for you to know is that your level of emotional support is highly critical. The more you are there for your partner; the better your relationship will be after the childbirth. The things you say to her **especially matter** while she is becoming increasingly more troubled by her body's transformation.

Let's say you find it increasingly humorous that she is getting larger and larger. You might say something like, "You look like a whale." Now most women are not going to appreciate your humor, they are going to think, "What a jerk!"

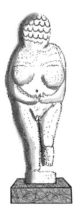 Now if by chance Phil said the right thing once during one of Genny's pregnancies. He happened to look at her when she was really large and her breasts were swollen and darkened. The thought went through his mind, "She looks like one of those fertility goddesses." But instead of saying that he realized that she wouldn't take it as just a comment that related to an interest in the anthropological aspects of birth. So then Phil thought to himself, "What can I say?" "Well," he said, "You are as womanly as you will ever be." Look, how much more feminine and full of life can a woman be than to be fully ripe with a beautiful child in her womb? (Remember ancient civilizations adored, worshipped and sacrificed to this womanly image.) Today, Genny still brags about that comment.

Buried Land Mines

Emotions can be buried inside of us. We know that for us men, we are much better in understanding the actual functions of a jet engine than we are of emotions. Turbines make sense. Tears and expressions of emotion are just indistinct, unfathomable and plain awkward. Logic is stable; intuition is weird. We've learned that emotions are comparable to liquids in corked bottles. Pull the cork out and watch what pours out. Grief is a powerful emotion.

In Phil's own life he has found that when one of his friends shared with him that they had a scary chronic illness, that he just felt this overwhelming sense of grief – like they had just died or something else terrible. In going through those emotions, he realized that his soul was also struggling more than it should. The grief we felt was coming from something more than that simple private disclosure. In examining his own feelings, he suddenly understood that he was grieving for another friend's recent tragedy. Remember when emotions aren't dealt with in our lives they become bottled up inside of us. Then, when one pricks the surface of our heart by introducing another emotionally charged issue, a whole supercharged lot may come out.

Now, let's say your relationship with your partner is still fresh. Or let's say things just never came up. You may find the pregnancy and birth experience a place where there can be some surprises. Then even more perplexing is when the heightened emotional state of pregnancy exposes something you thought was uncovered and dealt with. Whatever the case, there can be some scary moments that expose the inner soul of your partner.

Different vulnerabilities may come forth. If your partner has withheld information from you in fear that you might reject her, such as the past relationships she has had, and the possibility of previous births, abortions, sexual abuse, incest, or a myriad of other deep and dark secrets, you may find you are in shock, or you may be offended or hurt that these things weren't ever brought up. You may think you know everything about your partner, but birth can pull these closeted skeletons out into the bright sunshine.

Be very careful at how your respond to any of these. You may have some extraordinary emotions about the disclosure. You need to keep focused and produce as much positive support as possible. These confessions require nothing more than a listening ear. The more one exposes one's soul to another, the stronger the bonds of love will grow. However if you react in a non-supportive way, you may find ethereal love squandered for naught.

Shame, guilt, bitterness and other emotions just need a sympathetic ear. Emotions don't need fixing. Remember you can do nothing more with liquid than to contain it, freeze it or vaporize it. A healthy soul is one that learns how to control the emotions well enough to free them up in a non-hurtful way. If your mission is to provide the safest environment for the mother to have a child and a loving home for the child, then your control of your responses will have major impact.

Defusing the Duds

Some of these explosives you will find need serious defusing. Incest and sexual abuse can cause some women to want to shut down sexually, and this will affect her ability to land the baby -- to give birth. Apparently the psychology of birth

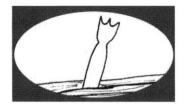

requires a woman to want to have the baby, to want to birth it -- to help cultivate a safe and effective birth process.

Just think if you were a woman who had been abused sexually by your father or relative. You might tell yourself that you never want to have a baby ever. You may say that to yourself until your brain is certain of its truth.

Many say that half of all women have in some way been sexually violated. Birth and pregnancy can bring out some of these forgotten or suppressed memories. Some warning signs that your partner may have been sexually abused include the following:

- Extreme need to control every aspect of the birth
- Extreme willingness to give up responsibility to others
- Feelings of great vulnerability
- Fear of dependency
- Confusion about sexuality
- Feeling unworthy or deserving of bad and painful events
- Extreme fear of being exposed (nakedness)
- Avoidance of male caregivers
- Fears of medical tests

Disarming bombs is dangerous. People get killed. Some women don't want their past lives revisited. They have buried their emotions under piles of concrete. They may have built a super powerful shield to keep others away. Your partner may have a deadly bomb down in her heart. You may try to reach out to help unbury this bomb, but encourage her to see the appropriate help – there are people who trained to detonate emotional bombs and you aren't the one. Remember you can't fix anyone emotionally. Love is acceptance. Just be warned that pregnancy can uncover hidden and powerful emotions.

Awareness does not change the heart. Some people are held in their fears or operate comfortably under delusions. The idea here is to understand that as a navigator you must protect your partner and make her feel loved, desired, cherished and supported. Attacking a lie that someone has held on to since childhood is serious psychological warfare. People sometimes will even tell you that their lie is part of their personality and that they like that part, because it protects them. The men who have violated these women didn't protect them, so they created an impenetrable hide. Often these women have strong wills and amazing determination. Don't stand in their way, just recognize that pregnancy and birth shake up their world and sometimes these misconceptions and falsehoods come into contact with reality. When an emotional wound is touched upon, resist the desire to remove the roots. Just let the pain ooze out -- that is healing enough. Just don't walk into this childbirth and pregnancy unaware of how intense things may become.

Agreement Is Everything

Long before your partner is in labor, strive to know her better. Listen a lot even if you don't understand all the emotions that pour forth. Stand there and enjoy the rain. These tears, these fears, these hurts and pains, they are intimacy. They join the minds and souls of two made one. The more you understand your partner and the more you can agree upon, the stronger you are together. The real bonds of love are commitment, acceptance and vulnerability.

A Wing Man Never Leaves His Post!

When you do not turn away under fire, you are a hero, no matter what the circumstance. The whole focus of a marital vow is to say you will stick it out through sickness and health, good times or bad times. Heading into the unknown territory of birth, you go in understanding that hell or high water you will do everything in your power to never let your captain down. You fly knowing that death could be around the corner, and you fly with determination.

We are men. We are the strong, the proud, and the brave. Men are born for adversity, to handle extreme pressure. Outside of actual warfare, childbirth may present the most difficult of emotional experiences for us. But, if we are prepared, we are able to overcome. Just look at all our own fathers—they survived didn't they. Who knows, the child coming to you may be the next Rembrandt, George Washington Carver, or John F. Kennedy.

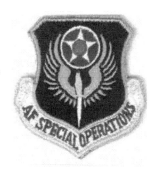

All of us have faced times in our lives when we wanted to bail out. Courage is facing the troubles of life. Cowardice is checking out and abandoning your post. Who hasn't felt like packing it in? Birth can shake up your world too, but the brave are able to hang in there. **A wingman never leaves his post.**

Promoting Positive Emotions

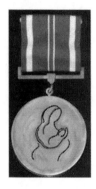

Helping your partner believe in herself, and her body's design, is something that any birth professional should be working toward, and you should join that effort. If she knows that relaxation helps reduce pain, but doesn't believe she is capable of relaxing, then there is a problem. A study shows that the more confident a woman is the better. So if you don't believe, then you can negatively affect your partner. It's like a faith thing. Most women are not prepared for the pain associated with their first childbirth experiences, and so much of handling childbirth is handling the uncomfortable stress, weight and pain. Having a partner who is confident about her ability to deal with all that is essential. Much of what doctors and midwives do is to help a woman deal with the pain. Birth techniques all seem to revolve around this idea. So try your best in encouraging your partner to believe in herself and in the natural design of her body. Remember every woman deserves an award for carrying children.

Celebrating

Baby showers are the main place where women celebrate pregnancy and birth. This is vitally important to your partner. You really shouldn't get involved with planning such an event, but you may be very sorry if you don't guarantee someone out there is going to take the time to plan one for her. The effects of not having a baby shower could impact your partner detrimentally. If your partner is not in a place where she has

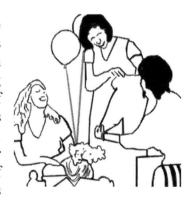

women in her life who will help her with this at the beginning of the pregnancy, you may want to try and get her connected socially (it is a misnomer that we as adults don't need others).

Social places like gyms, children's play groups, religious organizations, etc. are great places for your partner to make those connections, but it becomes very difficult for a shower to happen if you have recently moved to a new city and away from your partner's normal social group. The women in your partner's close social group are the ones that will pull off such an event. Yet since most often guys are excluded in a shower situation, we don't even think about this. Just try to celebrate her pregnancy with her in some way.

Another important celebration that should be handled is the arrival. Often people send cards and flowers and gifts at the baby's arrival – it is the first birthday party. You should realize the importance this event has. Many of us grew up in homes where there was little celebration at our birthdays. This is too bad. Everyone should be celebrated. Therefore make sure the birthday has its celebration. You can help coordinate this, but it usually happens spontaneously. However, you should at least go out and buy something for the new baby. If you don't have a car seat, that is a must, but it really isn't thoughtful. Depending on the season, you might think about buying a special blanket or outfit to handle the weather. Our oldest son was born in the dead cold of winter (it took about an hour to warm up the car for the drive home). Also when an athlete or beauty queen wins the contest, they receive a garland or flowers as tokens of appreciation. Most people never express the joy and satisfaction towards the mother and just focus on the child that was born, leaving the mother feeling out of place and not celebrated. So don't forget to honor the mother with some tribute to her success.

Again, just as in the baby shower, the birthday must be celebrated. The richer the celebration, often the better the woman will feel. However, remember that if your partner's experience was negative, even a good birthday party will not take away her emotional pain – which is sometimes supplemented by physical pain especially after a surgery. The classic song's lyrics ring true "It's my party and I'll cry if I want to!" As in all things regarding birth, try to understand what your captain is feeling and fit into her world to support her.

Emotional Territory

Birth is probably the most intense emotional experience your partner will ever have in her life. Making the experience positive is the goal you should have for her. When we take in an event and replay it later on in our lives, we remember it emotionally. This is ever true for birth. Women will either feel joy and triumph forever more about their birth experience or they could walk away with a feeling of defeat, hurt and violation. Since you are associated directly with this experience, you will forevermore be connected to this event as well, so the better the outcome the better your place in your partner's emotional memory of life. Women describe their birth experiences eons later with full emotion – tears streaming or with their faces beaming. The poetic echoes of birth never stop sounding. If you've experienced a traumatic birth, there are certain steps you can take to alleviate or resolve some of the disappointment that occurred during a crash landing. We will present ideas for doing a re-do later in Chapter 18.

Phil has heard women speak about what a loser their partner was at the birth, and how they would never want their partner to attend another birth. He was surprised that some of these women even want to bear another child. Yet if your partner has a bad experience, she may turn around and want to produce another child to queue up another birth where she can come out a winner. It's as if the prize is not the baby but rather the experience of the birth. You could compare it to a carnival game of knocking down the ten cans with two beanbags. You only get three throws per game. Many times because of interference, a woman may feel like she almost got them all down, and she could taste it. This is probably the psychology behind those stupid games – you keep paying until you get all the cans down. After one bad birth experience, women often either rise to the occasion or retreat. This may even affect their desire to have sexual relations. Irrationality may arise if she fears getting pregnant again. Makes sense doesn't it. If you just had a traumatic experience, you may avoid all resemblance of what put you in the position in the first place. That is why educating yourself and your partner on the first go around is important.

Postpartum Depression & Its Prevention

This is a state where a woman perceives that she had no control over her birth, she feels in despair and helpless. This is especially true when a woman has a desired expectation such as having a natural childbirth. When women go into the hospital and don't have adequate support, they may expect to have a nice uncomplicated birth. But this has very small chance of happening. The birth machine and the technocratic philosophy of birth have a high occurrence of interventions, surgeries and higher levels of neonatal and perinatal death. So many women's expectations are dashed. They want birth to be a certain way, but life doesn't always go as expected. What is of significance is that women who whole heartily buy into the technocratic birth idea and feel in control of the birth machine, they don't have any issues with depression. Depression comes from setting up an expectation and missing the mark wide.

It is the expectation and the feeling of control that is at issue. You may want the best for your partner, but she is the only one who will have in her mind the conceptual birth she wants – if that doesn't happen **you both may suffer trauma**. As mentioned, divorce and breakup are part of the effects of childbirth. A study, funded by the National Institutes of Health at Texas A&M, was called *The effect of the transition to parenthood on relationship quality: An eight- year prospective study*, and found that up to 90% of couples reported dissatisfaction in their relationships after the birth of their first child. It doesn't have to be that way. According to Alyson Fearnley Shapiro and Dr. John Gottman authors of the study, *The baby and the marriage: Identifying factors that buffer against decline in marital satisfaction after the first baby arrives*, out of University of Washington , the three-part prescription for strengthening the relational bonds includes (1) Building fondness and affection for your partner; (2).Being aware of what is going on in your spouse's life and being responsive to it; and (3) Approaching problems as something you and your partner can control and solve together as a couple.

Aligning yourself means you should not put yourself at odds with your partner and that you should learn what her expectations are, and help to ensure that she has the birth she wants. However, if you partner wants a natural childbirth and has a lot in common with the holistic approach, and she is in the hospital, then there is a huge problem. You are under the domain of the hospital, and so those expectations are excruciatingly hard to see happen. Some will tell you that the hospital is the most sterile place, but that isn't actually true, not that everyone's home is cleaner. The point is that if your partner feels safer and more serene in the hospital for birthing a child then that is where you should support her going.

The emotional impact of childbirth is unlike any other interaction you will have with your partner. The body produces certain opiates naturally while the labor is progressing. If you are there and you are seen as part of a good experience, her thoughts of you will be highly positive, but if you are distant and not part of the process, you may be viewed negatively. If you have an opposite point of view during the process, you may even be seen as an enemy. You want to be the protector here, the one helping your partner get what she needs out of her birth – not just the baby but the birth experience.

Once a woman has a negative experience, you may find that she turns more towards either the technocratic, birth machine, mentality, or she may go in the opposite direction. Some women believe that the machine was right in tearing them up with their interventions, and these women may even go back to support that model. Other women may go back to their doctors and demand a change if they get pregnant again. A bad outcome will cause internal conflicts within these women, and they often go well beyond expectations. Women have formed organization, started schools, become childbirth educators, become La Leche Leaders, etc. Birth has a power of transforming lives, and when one is dissatisfied with their experience they either stay depressed or promote some type of change.

In reading many birth stories for the writing of this book, we were amazed at the diversity of how women make their decisions. Sometimes women who had a nasty birth in the birth machine turn around and schedule themselves for planned cesarean sections the second go around. Sometimes a woman who had a tough natural delivery will chose to have their next baby with every possible intervention – especially those used to cut the intensity of pain. Some women just get more empowered and go back at the birth machine better prepared to hold off the interventions. Others have decided that they want to have the babies at home without any midwife or doctor. Men need to realize their place, and that place is not always the same. We all will not make the same choice. Since the woman is like the football team captain, we just run the play that is called to the best of our abilities. She is the captain.

You need to do what is best for your partner (for that is what is good for you), and that is why you need to know her well. Knowing her birth philosophy and affirming it is essential. Both of you need to get that done well before you start the labor.

Intelligent Communications

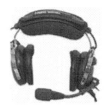

Since birth is a huge test on your relationship with your captain, you need to implement an effective communication strategy. This means you think ahead of time and plan how you can be involved with this birth, and to communicate how you are going to be supportive of your partner. She needs for you to come to the birth with an attitude of consensus and agreement. She needs to know that you are there and that you will accommodate her plan.

This means that you must communicate well and even put it down in writing, so as to have a place of complete understanding. Disappointment comes from having a false expectation. Even simple things can become a big problem, especially when there are false assumptions. Don't assume you are understood or that you've understood her. The more detail orientated your partner is, the more detailed her plan might end up.

In all communication training, there is the two-way diagram. This means you have two parties who have to send and receive messages. If your message is vague or unclear, your partner may just get the wrong message. Ask your partner questions allowing for her point of view to be heard.

Communications with the Birth Team

Depending on whom you are working with, you will find different levels of communications with the folks helping you with this birth. You need to be effectively communicating with these people. Several issues come to mind. If you find that the birth team communicates to you and your partner that you have no say or autonomy in your coming birth, you need to stand up for your partner. This experience is yours first and foremost. They may deliver thousands of babies, but, as it is your children, you get only a few births in your life. So the power struggle between those who come to birth as if it were to be managed by the specialists and that you are just a subordinate and that you should keep quiet and out of the way. That means when you get into this, and select your birth team, you should work with those who understand your point of view.

Laws, Regulations, Etc.

We live in a litigious society. We have laws about medicine and health. You need to learn all you can about what regulations and laws are in effect. Oftentimes, hospitals will have a rights document. There is a big advocacy push in our country to provide that we as patients have rights. You need to have those rights in mind when you enter someone else's territory.

At home you have freedom and require no rights document. The hospital environment is designed for the institution's convenience, that's why you need rights. For normal births, a home is often the safest place to be since you control the territory. When birth deviates from the normal pattern and there are indications of a possible poor outcome, then transfer to the hospital is appropriate.

In the hospital you may risk being put on the surgery mass production line. The machine just spits out babies. You may be fencing every minute with staff trained to follow the machine's dictates. The birth interventions may take over if you don't police what is happening – or have a Doula or birth assistant helping. It can be like a runaway train.

However, insisting that nothing goes wrong and willfully stopping a transfer to the hospital can result in just as bad of a birth as the interventionary doctors. So if you stay in the home, know that you should trust the wisdom and experience of your practitioners.

Remember the whole point in this thing is to land the plane safely with that precious cargo undamaged.

Knowing the laws of the community you live in helps you have a voice in the hospital and the ability to transfer there if you decide to have a home birth and a transfer results. You need to be equipped either way to deal with that. If you live in a jurisdiction where midwifery is still illegal, the doctors may prosecute your home practitioner if they find out that you were trying to birth at home. For some places midwifery is outlawed and the medical establishment has a virtual monopoly. Some doctors in this country form a very powerful and financially well-stocked lobby that still oppose midwifery.

Aggressive Communication

When and if you have to communicate with anyone involved in birth, you need to learn to reduce or eliminate aggressive communication patterns. This is not a very easy thing to do especially in the culture or competition and aggression, which we men have grown up with. Many techniques exist to improve our ways of speaking so as to improve our ability to share our needs and to learn of our partner's needs thus improving our chances of having those needs met.

Fear and Control

What we have learned most about women in general is that the more empowered they feel the more they will make decisions regarding their births. In an article titled "The Effect of Prenatal Education on Beliefs/Perceptions" it was clear that the level of fear in women was reduced when they took prenatal classes and that those who wanted to actively participate in the birth had increases in their desire to do so. When women are not encouraged to be actively involved many become helpless, dependent, and terribly afraid of childbirth. Childbirth education classes help women perceive that they have control over the event, reducing their fear. By being autonomous, informed and making her own decisions, a woman becomes empowered. The data suggest that this is a way for her to overcome the fear of childbirth.

Chapter 6: Morale

Involvement means encouragement. Whatever you can do to involve yourself with your partner's pregnancy, it is for the better. You need to know that every minute you devote to this special time is encouraging to your partner, and that facilitates a protected environment for the baby's development. It's like you are preparing a protected base camp ahead of the coming troops. Everything you do is furthering a feeling of security and strength. This is how you can build your partner's confidence. Every little thing you do will help provide a haven of peace and serenity. Research reveals that the more involved you are after the pregnancy is confirmed, the more active and enthusiastic you will be as a father. Good fathers are in short supply.

Primary Source Encouragement

Several simple and commonsensical areas need to be encouraged as soon as you know your partner is pregnant. You need to promote your partner's actions. She needs to eat healthy foods. She needs to get ample exercise. She needs sleep. Then, as much as possible, you should help to provide a stress-free environment. Further she needs adequate and immediate prenatal care. These are things she should be doing, but she may not be. Pregnancy can bring about a lot of awkwardness for a woman especially if this is her first baby and/or if she wasn't expecting a baby. Your solid support of the coming child and the encouragement you give your mate will influence them greatly. She may think that a child is an imposition on your relationship – prove otherwise. For her health and the child's health, these kinds of thoughts need to be dealt with and hopefully laid to rest. Vulnerability is huge at this time. By stepping in and taking away her fears, you will be conquering the worst enemy of human existence: fear.

If you have gotten off to a bad start, and you have a great deal of apprehension and fear yourself, then keep that negativity away from the mother and coming child. Take it to counseling, journal it, or whatever it takes. Unkind words and careless deeds reflect an immature relationship. Stay off that course. This is not the time to say harsh things. Words are painful and will affect the mother and the child. The baby needs positive words and needs to be welcomed. This is your child, so you need to control your tongue and extinguish any temper you may have. Think of how you would treat a newborn child – gently and with tenderness. That is how you should treat your partner if you truly love her. Stick to this type of attitude, and you are sure to improve your relationship beyond compare.

If you get angry easily, you need to learn some anger management techniques before you get to the big event. First, you do not control anything, or anyone, but yourself. So do that, control yourself. If you get peeved, walk away from the situation or person, and if that is your partner during the birth, tell her you are taking a break and will be back – but don't tell her you are upset with her, she needs to focus on the job at hand and not on your feelings.

Creative Flight

Pregnancy is a time like no other. It is a time of growth development, change and creativity. A couple may tap into this creative power of new growth and create new and lasting lifestyle changes for everyone's betterment. A typical pregnancy lasts around nine months, and that is ample time to see improved habits form. The pregnancy provides the pallet to draw upon to create vibrant choices for the refining of one's health. Pregnant couples have not only nurtured and developed a child throughout the pregnancy, but many have renewed comments to a closer and more intimate relationship, they have instituted campaigns for regular and more meaningful exercise and communication. They have overhauled their eating habits to support the development of the new life their union has created and thus improved their own eating habits. They have taken up new hobbies, learned new games or skills. We encourage you to capture all the positive energy that your pregnancy is offering to you and your mate to set a course for sustained lifetime changes. Take these nine months and mine them for all the gems that this precious season has to offer. There are so many arenas that you and your partner may explore that can be enriched and enhanced by the pregnancy experience. Take stock and think about what you both want to change in your lives and do it.

Human Touch

As men, we are not too touchy. One of the most effective means of encouraging a woman is to touch her. We men fail miserable at that. During pregnancy and especially during a labor and delivery, touch is a powerful way of encouraging your partner. Recent studies have shown that male partners are much less likely to touch a laboring partner than a female Doula or labor assistant. Touch reassures a woman. It provides a physical communication of love and support. It would benefit all men to learn to touch their partners with a gentle, non-sexual touch. This would improve your ability to be there for your partner, and it would improve the probability of the type of outcome we all want. So touch her. That's right stroke her. Massage her. Hold her close. Anything but sit there like a cold statue. If you can't do it, then pay for someone who will.

Mess Hall

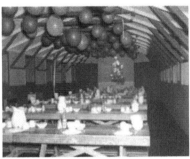

As we have discussed in the section on physiological changes, a mother needs to eat a whole lot to grow a baby. You can help her by preparing foods that you know will nourish the mother and baby. You can ensure healthy eating by eating that way as well. Whatever the mother ingests will affect the baby's development. A diet that is rich in essential nutrients is essential.

By the fourth month of pregnancy, a woman needs to eat around 500 more calories per day. But all through the pregnancy it is important to eat quality nutritious foods. The traditional three meals a day doesn't work well for pregnancy, and as the baby grows, the intestines and stomach cannot accommodate that level of food in the digestive track. Your partner may need more like 6 to 8 meals. Preparing healthy snacks, sandwiches and soups are a good idea to provide plenty to eat, but also make sure that that plenty is healthy and nutritious. Fresh fruits and vegetables contain an abundance of vitamins that are needed in this process. You may find the pregnancy helps to improve your own diet as well.

Your partner may find milk a very good source of Vitamins A and D. Cheese is a substitute as well as yogurt. Potatoes with their skins can be baked and provide calcium, iron, protein, thiamine, riboflavin, niacin and a good amount of Vitamin C. Without the skins, you lose a great deal of their best stuff, so shun the fried or peeled. You may need to alter food selections if there are food allergies -- a common one being lactose-intolerant, so milk may not always be a good food.

Avoid foods that have their nutrients either reduced or destroyed by canning, pasteurizing or freezing. Foods with extra preservatives or artificial coloring or flavorings contain chemicals that are unneeded and undesirable. Excess sugar or carbohydrates from white flour products add little nutrition and contain "empty" calories. Strong coffee and the tannic acid in tea are not good. The acid can stop the absorption of iron, and caffeine in large quantities has a negative effect on the developing child. Soda has both the empty calories and often caffeine, so it should also be avoided.

Simple steps can be taken to enrich the nutrient content of dietary choices that you already enjoy. Bread and cereal selection can increase the amount of protein you take in simply by making the choice of a higher protein content bread or cereal. The same holds true with yogurt and cheeses. Enjoy marketing together and evaluate the nutritional contents listed on the food labels of comparable meal items. Make a game of it and see who can pack the cart with the highest protein count. Get the most bang for your buck when it comes to foods and purchase and eat **nutrient dense** foods. You dietary selections should pack proteins, minerals and vitamins.

Vital Nutrients

Most often the health care practitioner will make sure that your partner is taking a prenatal vitamin. This issue of proper nutrition has the ability to affect the developing child and can even cause low birth weight or premature labor. A woman's protein intake needs to increase by 50% during the pregnancy. Vegetable proteins cannot provide the proper types of amino acids so they should be combined with animal protein of some type. Of course protein can be found in peas, lentils, seeds, nuts, etc. Fiber is important to avoid the "all too common" constipation. As mentioned earlier, just as there is a need to increase the calories, there is an equal need to increase the liquid intake. As a matter of fact, proteins require even more liquid for absorption in your partner's system.

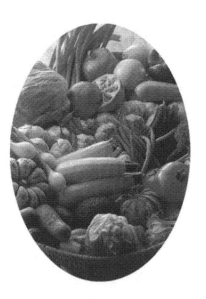

Minerals are also a big part of keeping your partner's body healthy during a pregnancy. Magnesium is required at rates of 450 mgs per day when most people intake only 160 to 260 mgs (milligrams) per day. Whole grains, leafy greens, nuts and tofu are a good source. Maternal hemorrhaging is lessened in women who take supplements of this mineral.

Calcium supplements are helpful if you buy the type that dissolve (to test place tablet in a cup of room temperature vinegar – stir vigorously every five minutes – if the tablet doesn't dissolve in 30 minutes you need a better supplement. Food like milk and cheese are fine if your partner can handle the lactic sugar – some adults are allergic to it. Calcium is important for forming the baby's bodies, reducing the erosion of the maternal skeletal system, and helps reduce hypertension in women.

With the blood volume up so high, women need more iron. However, the most common iron supplement is ferrous sulfate – this type of supplement is known to cause constipation. Floradix, an iron syrup supplement is recommended but ferrous fumarate and gluconate are all right. Many recommend that iron is taken with orange juice to help in absorption. Note that some minerals and vitamins tend to cause nausea in the first trimester. Dosages over 30 milligrams are not recommended as they tend to interfere with the absorption of other nutrients.

Fueling Growth

A woman's needs for energy, protein, water, vitamins and minerals all increase to meet the needs of the developing baby and the many changes the mother's body undergoes. During the second and third trimesters of pregnancy a woman's need for calories increases. A pregnant woman needs an additional 25 grams of protein per day above the needs of a non-pregnant woman. This additional protein is necessary for the development of the placenta, breasts, and uterus, and as well as for the construction of the baby itself.

With the increase of blood volume and the manufacturing of the amniotic fluid, there consequently is a need for additional water. Drinking more water is also relevant in preventing constipation. We all can benefit from drinking more water. It is recommended that a woman drink about 2 liters of water per day during pregnancy (Smolin & Grosvenor 2003). B vitamins, thiamin, niacin, and riboflavin, B6, zinc, calcium, vitamins C and D, folate vitamin B12 and Iron are all needed in greater amounts during pregnancy to achieve protein synthesis of the new cells necessary in fetal and maternal tissues. These micronutrients provide for the new growth and development of bones and connective tissue in addition to the formation of new maternal and fetal cells.

Turbulence: Common Discomforts of Pregnancy

As you and your mate go on this flight you may experience some turbulence on your flight pattern. 50% of all pregnancies are accompanied by morning sickness, the nausea and vomiting that women wake up to in the early weeks of pregnancy. This nausea is attributed to the rising hormone levels in the mother. It takes some time for her body to acclimate to these rising levels. Genny would add right here and now that the reason it is called morning sickness is because you wake up with it in the morning, and it is still there from yesterday. The idea that morning sickness is only in the hours upon waking is a misnomer. Some foods to contend with Morning Sickness are suggested by Middleton and Rapitis in their excellent book <u>The Healthy Pregnancy Cookbook</u>. They recommend ginger tea, gingerale, crackers, toast, rice, skinless chicken and turkey breasts and plain noodles just to mention a few. On the positive side of morning sickness, studies demonstrate that the more acute the morning sickness the greater likelihood that the pregnancy will continue to term. This does not mean that if you are fortunate enough not to experience morning sickness that the pregnancy will be miscarried.

For the first several weeks of pregnancy while hormones level out for smooth flight the woman's body undergoes major physiological changes. Fatigue often accompanies the early months of pregnancy. Frequently this fatigue like no other does lighten up towards the middle of pregnancy. In flight the highest amount of fuel load is utilized in just getting the plane off the ground, and we can liken the first trimester to the plane taking off and getting airborne. When the placenta is developing and the baby is taking form, it reflects the efforts needed to retrofit a design of an air craft to carry a special payload. Women get exhausted from this physical work. Once airborne, the energy requirements adjust for maintaining the flight. Pregnancy is similar in that women have at least the better part of 3 months to create the life support (the placenta) and the baby, and once these are firmly established the flight levels out until it is time to approach for landing.

Remember she may also be irritable and cranky in this productive state. Think about having thrown up for three weeks straight and not being able to keep anything down.

The discomforts of pregnancy, physically and emotionally (forgetfulness, bouts of tears, emotional highs and lows), are all related to the changing physiology and increased hormone levels of pregnancy -- particularly progesterone. We cannot emphasis enough the importance of good nutrition in maintaining well-being in pregnancy. Making nutrient rich dietary choices supports the body through the many stresses of pregnancy, and also diminishes many discomforts. There is a reference chart included for you in the appendices that provides information about the more common discomforts of pregnancy and what can be done to alleviate them.

Camp Exercise

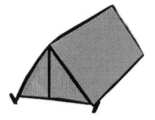

Women still need exercise to be as healthy as possible. The better condition your partner is in the greater chance that she will be able to handle the event of birth that requires physical endurance. However, you should ensure your partner avoids exercise that may cause falling, jarring and joint stress such as horseback riding, skiing, surfing, and contact and racquet sports. Even bike riding can be problematic after a certain point. Just have her use commonsense when walking, swimming, or doing aerobics, etc. Avoid anything that jerks the body and could jerk the uterus. You may find like we have that walking in a comfortable pair of shoes or going swimming are the best forms of exercise. Swimming is the best form of exercise during pregnancy because the buoyancy in water accommodates the physical changes of the pregnant body.

Pregnant women should check with their health care providers when taking on exercise programs. Women who were physically exercising before their pregnancy should be encouraged to continue, and women who have not exercised before their pregnancy may begin an exercise campaign remembering to start slowly with low impact. As we have mentioned earlier pregnancy can provide the catalyst for inspiring a healthier lifestyle.

It is important for the mother not to become overheated when exercising to prevent inadequate delivery of oxygen and nutrients to the baby. Intense exercise should be kept to a minimum and the woman should be drinking plenty of fluids. The exercise environment should be adequately ventilated.

You may encourage your partner by participating. Long walks are very refreshing and provide a goodly amount of exercise. They are also very emotionally reassuring to your partner – and can be quite romantic. Stay positive and talk about things especially if they are the positive energy types of subjects that make one smile.

Weight Gain

Pregnant women need to focus on eating balanced diets, and not be so concerned about weight gain. The average woman who gains between 25 and 35 pounds is more apt to have a healthy baby of normal weight. A pregnant woman's weight gain fluctuates and has a lot to do with whether a woman has morning sickness. However, the guidelines are for about one pound per week during the second and third trimesters. Overweight women are recommended to gain half that much. However, if a woman goes into the pregnancy overweight, and she eats extremely well, she may gain little weight and get into better health during her pregnancy. We had personal experience with this with during the pregnancy of our fourth child. Yes, a woman can change her lifestyle and habits during a pregnancy.

Scientists studying pregnancy and weight gain found that thin women that gain weight also find that their babies gain proportionally while that is not true for overweight women. So with a thin woman the weight recommendation may have more relevance.

Although we will share with you the common guidelines regarding weight gain in pregnancy, one needs to be open the individuality of the course of weight gain during a pregnancy. Naturally a woman who enters her pregnancy underweight will need a greater degree of weight gain to support the pregnancy. Genny is living proof that a woman who enters a pregnancy in less than a ideal weight with wise nutritional choices and adequate exercise actually may develop a healthy infant and come out on the other side of the pregnancy in better physical shape than before the pregnancy began. We enjoyed watching this magnificent transformation of Genny's health throughout our last pregnancy.

Generally speaking with the development of the baby, placenta, amniotic fluid and additional maternal blood, fluid and tissue necessary to support the pregnancy a (typical) woman is looking at a weight gain of between 25- 35 lbs. It is fascinating what the body goes thru to support a pregnancy.

Development	Amount
Baby	7-8 lbs
Amniotic Fluid	2 lbs
Placenta	1-2 lbs
Uterus	2 lbs
Increase in Mother's Blood Volume	3-4 lbs
Increase in Breast Tissue	2 lbs
Additional Cellular Fluids	4 lbs
Additional Maternal Fat	4-11 lbs
Total Weight Gain	25-35 lbs

Medic Visits

Prenatal care is a very good way to foster the best possible health of mother and child. As a man you may not feel the need to be there for those appointments, but it should be something you place in the category of encouraging. You want to go to the first prenatal appointment. It's like having someone come to your first performance or to your first ball game. Don't leave your mother-to-be alone. She may not seem to need much more support or encouragement, but this first appointment means a lot. Be there for her. This sets the tone for the birth team.

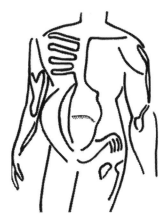

If you intend to be at the birth, you need to know everyone who is going to be there, and you need to know their roles and responsibilities, as well as they need to know where you fit. You don't want to let your partner down by not involving yourself in the planning or the rehearsals. Take the whole day off and go with your partner to some of these appointments. Take her out to eat, and make it a surprise.

Prenatal appointments are scheduled every four weeks until the 28th week. After that, until week 36, the schedule is every two weeks. Finally from the 36th week until the birth, the appointments are weekly. That gives you plenty of time to plan on attending some of these prenatals with your partner.

Uniforms Changes

During the first part of a pregnancy, your partner will not need anything special as far as clothing, but that is a good time to buy some clothing for the larger shape your partner will take. Let her make the choices, but make it an outing – as much as most of us hate shopping. The idea is to make her feel like a queen for the day. Honor here is important. You are honoring the sacred office of mother. Then remember to continue that routine each year at Mother's Day. Honor this most significant of events. This is the big one besides marriage and death. This is one of those huge events that most guys don't really comprehend. This is winning Wimbledon, the Super Bowl, the Series!

Now the point we're making here is that the change of shape your partner is going through must be honored. She is going to stretch and grow well beyond believability. Never say anything that doesn't honor this. She is being put through an ordeal physically to bring forth child, which can even in our technologically advanced day end badly. Your partner may to look at herself in the mirror when she gets really large. She's going to cry and say she is horrifically ugly. Put it this way, you can't go into that.

You can't risk your life to bring forth this baby. So just like you would highly honor the guy who jumps into the burning building to pull out your kids, honor her.

Clothing, jewelry, makeup, and all the fineries help her to see the best looking woman she can be. Encourage that. Then tell her how beautiful her developing body is and she'll still feel good about herself. That is our charge. Make your partner know without doubt that you confirm every change. Actually you should count pregnancy as a great honor in your life as well.

Establishing New Routines

After you have done all, enjoy the miracle of the baby's development. It is surely the most amazing biological happening you will be involved with. You should know that sometimes women get so caught up in this marvelous experience that they overlook you, so make the effort to set up a special time with your partner, for you as well as for her. Possible make it a routine to spend time each week learning about the various aspects of the baby's growth stages.

You can buy a book that has plenty of pictures and information about each of the stages: 1st trimester, etc. Usually these books will detail many of the amazing things science has learned about how a child grows. Routines are good to develop in any relationship, so take advantage of this time to institute a new event each week. Just like you may have a time to read together, go on a date, see a movie, or attend religious services. Setting a designated time to talk about this will only strengthen your relationship and you can keep yourself from being excluded. Plus, the facts are quite interesting to learn. Do you know when the baby first has fingers or eyelashes? After the pregnancy, you could extend that time to be a "discuss the baby" later to "family" time.

Lifestyle Choices: Tobacco & Alcohol

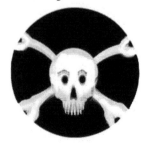

It should come as no big surprise that drugs, alcohol and cigarettes are not healthy to a developing child. If they can kill adults over prolonged use, or with overdoses, then they can only be harmful to a frail baby.

Studies show that ten cigarettes per day do in fact correlate to higher death levels of smokers' babies. Chemicals absorbed from smoke directly interfere with the growth of a baby. Carbon monoxide levels are much higher in the baby than the mother, and this is *poison*. Congenital defects are much higher in smokers' offspring. If you smoke and so does your partner, try and eliminate this habit during the pregnancy; it's healthier for everyone involved. It is a well-known fact that smoking can be one of the hardest habits to eliminate, so ensuring you have a healthy baby may just be that motivation you need. Just think of the second hand smoke – do you want your children to inhale that?

Alcohol is also a poison and can damage a developing child or kill it if amounts are high. This is most critical during the first 6 to 12 weeks of the pregnancy. Schenker in *Fetal Alcohol Syndrome: Current Status of Pathogenesis* demonstrates the toxic effect of alcohol on the unborn child. When a pregnant woman consumes alcohol, what she has drank crosses the placenta and enters the fetal blood stream at the same level of alcohol concentration as what she herself receives as an full grown adult. No safe level of consumption exists – everything is potentially potent. If your partner consumes more than two drinks per day, there is a one in ten chance the baby will develop (FAS), Fetal Alcohol Syndrome. FAS can cause birth defects and cause a child to have lower intelligence. The more severe the FAS, the harder it is for the child to ever catch up. Binge drinking can cause the same damage. The babies born from alcoholic mothers are in significant jeopardy of being affected by FAS. Try and encourage your partner to avoid alcohol throughout the pregnancy.

Drugs

All other drugs are risks. It is proven that during the critical 6 to 12 week development stage that drugs can interfere with the baby's development. Drugs in combination with other drugs or even food substances can be harmful even if they are not in themselves harmful. The dangers inherent in drugs suggest that your partner needs to be communicating with her health care provider about any medications she may need. This includes aspirin and over-the-counter substances. Yes, your partner may require some drugs for chronic illnesses like diabetes, but those issues should have been addressed prior to the pregnancy; otherwise they should be dealt with immediately. Drugs legal or illegal have the likelihood to really curse a child's growth and health. Even Tylenol can cause damage to the baby's developing kidneys and liver. Encourage your partner to be in contact with a knowledgeable health care professional when it comes to using any drugs.

What goes into mom is the same thing that goes into baby, but because baby's developing systems cannot remove the poisons effectively, they can kill or maim.

Consumer Reports mentions the ten over the counter drugs that should be avoided during pregnancy on their web site at the following location:

http://www.consumerreports.org/health/prescription-drugs/10-over-the-counter-drugs-to-avoid-during-pregnancy/overview/10-over-the-counter-drugs-to-avoid-during-pregnancy-ov.htm

Environmental Hazards

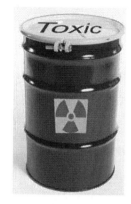

Outside of the consumption of drugs, you must be aware of serious problems with chemicals that can cause death to developing babies. We are talking about toxins and poisons that are found in all sorts of environments. Pesticides and other industrial chemicals, hydrocarbons, solvents, metals, oils, paints and lacquers, waste water treatment chemicals and other strong chemicals can kill. You know what we're talking about. We can't see a pregnant woman going out and tampering with these things, but you should be aware. Avoid strong glues, bleach, rubbing alcohol, ammonia and any other strong cleaners.

Cat Liter/Toxoplasmosis

Toxoplasmosis is an infection that is so mild to adults that they may not even notice the cold like symptoms that are associative with the infection. However this organism is extremely harmful to the unborn baby, causing malformations of the unborn baby to occur and even fetal death. Cats, especially cats that go outside and are hunters carry toxoplasmosis, and the organism can be found in the cats feces up to a year later. So, if you are the owner of a furry friend guys, you need to deal with the cat litter during the course of the pregnancy. It is a good idea to encourage the mother to wash her hands also after the handling of cats. Cats and their litter are not the only carriers of toxoplasmosis so are meats, that are not cooked thoroughly, and unwashed vegetables.

Saunas

Women who are pregnant need to be careful in their consideration of using a sauna or hot tub. Extremely high temperatures, such as can be found in saunas, can damage fetal development. Harvey et al. in a study "Suggested Limits to the Use of the Hot Tub and Sauna by Pregnant Women", in the Canadian Medical Association Journal July 1, 1981 sites "The high temperature of a fever may interfere with cell division and may cause birth defects or even fetal death if occurs repeatedly, for extended periods, or at a crucial time in fetal development." If the mother is an avid hot tub user, the temperature of the hot tub may be reduced to warm as opposed to hot, or she might limit her visits to the hot tub to only 10 minutes, it is unlikely that a temperature elevation should occur with a minimal time in the hot tub at reduced temperatures.

Fish Consumption

Fish is an excellent dietary choice packed with vital nutrients and omega oils, however the FDA has noted the concern regarding Mercury levels in fish especially for pregnant women. Mercury found in fish can affect the development of the baby's brain and nervous systems. The guidelines allow up to 12 ounces of low mercury fish, (Anchovies, Butterfish, Calamari (squid), Caviar (farmed), Crab (king) ,Pollock, Catfish, Whitefish, Perch (ocean), Scallops, Flounder, Haddock, Hake, Herring, Lobster (spiny/rock), Shad, Sole, Crawfish/crayfish, Salmon, Shrimp, Clams, Tilapia, Oysters, Sardines, Sturgeon (farmed) and Trout (freshwater) may be consumed weekly. These "high" level of mercury fish should be consumed at no more than 3 six ounce servings per month; Saltwater Bass, Croaker, Halibut, Tuna (canned, white albacore), Tuna (fresh Bluefin, Ahi), Sea Trout, Bluefish, and Lobster (American/Maine). Finally the FDA advises that those fish containing the highest levels of Mercury be avoided among those fish containing the highest level of mercury are; Grouper, Marlin, Orange Roughy, Tilefish, Swordfish, Shark, and Mackerel (king). The Natural Resources Defense Council (NRDC) maintains a list of fish and their current mercury levels, if you have questions regarding a fish that we have not mentioned here the council can provide the most current data on mercury levels of fish.

Chapter 7: The Territory of Birth

The Vision

Can you visualize what this pregnancy and birth are going to be like? Have you been through one of these missions before? Well, no matter what you visualize, every birth is a separate and individual event and one that you have only so much control over. However, don't lose heart, you can make a big difference in making decisions that will affect the birth – and that is your mission, to do everything within your power to guarantee that both mother and the developing child are cared for.

Simply speaking, your involvement must be in providing the best possible environment for the birth, and also in providing the best you have to offer in the pregnancy. Man's role covers three main areas: (a) you are the protector of the birth environment, (b) you are part of the emotional support, and (c) you are the father/guardian of the coming child. You need to learn about this mission to know what dangers really exist and when to intervene. You need to provide your partner as much emotional support as possible – which may also mean that you support others in providing that support. And, as the child coming is yours, you are the welcoming committee. Helping ensure your partner feels safe in having this child is probably the largest part of your whole mission. Succeed in that, and you most likely will have no trouble with the rest. Just think of it as providing a safe place for the flight and landing.

Since you are not a woman and never can truly understand what being one is like, just recognize that women need women in this process of birth. As we have it in us to want to protect others, they have it in them to nurture others. Your form of support is different. You become more of a rod of steel. You keep the peace and stop others from interfering.

Make sure that your partner is taken care of by people who will be nurturing especially if you are unable to muster much of that emotional support.

Mapping the Mission

In every childbirth education class we've been through, they tell you to prepare a birth plan. It is surprising how this little plan can affect the mission. When you look at writing down what you want to happen, be especially careful you don't go into too much detail. There have been studies that show that the longer and more complicated a plan is, the more likely for that plan to fail. How many times have we talked to someone who said that they had planned the birth a certain way only to have that come crashing down on their head? This was especially true if their expectations hit head on with a birth environment that took control of the birth.

Think about how you make plans. When describing how your next trip to the great outdoors, how detailed would you get? Frankly most of us just go about it without planning. Still writing down what you want to happen has a positive side. It makes you aware of what is forthcoming. It helps focus you on preparing properly. However, the more little details you chose to write down, the greater chance of you're missing the mark. The more marks you miss the greater chance of losing your focus, deflating your hopes.

Make your plan more like a game plan. You look over the situation and you call a few plays. You evaluate the opponents and pick out their strengths and weaknesses. A good wingman is going to have flexibility in their game plan. You only run the plan to help focus your efforts. During the mission all sorts of flexibility is needed. Just write down how you will approach the birth. This will help you gel with your partner and it will strengthen her feelings of support and security. The plan put together in unison should help bind you together as well.

Include Backup

Make sure you plan has built into it the landing and aftermath. Life is uncertain and unpredictable. You may have a clean easy landing. But all pilots are trained to make emergency landings. You birth planning should take into consideration events you don't want to see happening. You and your mate may end up having a child with a serious medical condition like a heart which requires surgery. It will hit you like your tires blow out on the airfield.

Our suggestion is that you include others in your planning. Make sure you have backup prepared to come in a help you through something unknowable. Let you care provider know about these backup people, by giving them instructions on who to call to get your team in gear. You should also have the backup team aware of what they can do to help you.

Hospitals will not have a place for parents of a sick child to stay. You back up team could support you by securing a hotel room near by. Meals might be needed. Your cat might need feeding, or your other children need running to school or having a care taker.

Look for those who make it their mission to support you. Family may be around to call upon, but for mobile Americans, you may have to develop a stronger social network – something men are notorious at not doing. Talk to friends and acquaintances or to the church. You might be surprised at who will enlist. Childbirth is to be celebrated by them as well, but if things go awry then they can stop a disaster from wiping out you and your family. All three of you need this built into your birth plan.

Choosing the Environment

In our experience environment is everything in birth. We all have seen women delivering their babies in taxis due to the fascination Hollywood has for awkward and unusual birth scenes. They want to throw in the extraordinary to bring out the drama. There are many comic birth scenes in the movies, and they are all worth laughing over. But picking out the right environment for birth is a something you and your partner should be serious about.

Remember the environment you chose can decide the fate of the mission. In our experience, if you have little control over the environment, your ability to create psychological tranquility is lost. It is a lot like choosing the set for a movie. Pick a set that engenders confidence and peace and serenity, if that is the landing you want.

What factors are there in selecting the most desired environment? This may have a lot to do with you and your partner's birth philosophy. Make sure you communicate with her about this. Many men think that birth is only a women's thing, and that they really don't want to volunteer. "Birth is women's work only!" is the prevalent attitude.

You should really want to protect your partner so that childbirth is a good experience and not one that is terrifying. This is huge. This will affect you, the child and the mother for the rest of your natural lives. You want that child to come into this world with as little trauma as possible. It should be your desire that the mother feels satisfied with her birth experience and that she will not look back at this as the most disappointing thing that ever happened to her.

There is a lot going on here. Think about this. First your partner has a mind, soul and body. The baby is not in her control. Her uterus is not in her control. The more she tries to control it, the most possibility she will have of upsetting the natural workings of her design. The more she let's go and can just let the process happen, to go inside herself and release her will, the easier for a birth to happen smoothly. Women can go into a labor, and then either interrupt themselves or be interrupted by others and then the process shuts down.

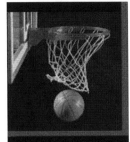

We as men can understand a little of what it is like to let loose and give over to our natural abilities when we think about sports. The more we think about how to do something that requires coordination and timing, the more likely we will freeze up. Sports require us to just shoot the jumper at the buzzer, not think about it. We need to relax our minds to let the mechanics of a certain silky stroke or awesome athletic maneuver to happen effortlessly. That is why we play our best when we are in the best environments, and sometimes under the most pressure.

Hospitals

Most people choose the hospital for their birth mainly because the medical profession operates in that environment, because their insurance pays for it, and because North Americans have been taught that birth is only safe in a hospital where all the emergency equipment is. Since most of births in the U.S., occur in this environment or territory, people assumed you should have your baby there.

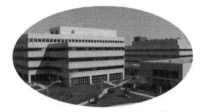

Good reasons for choosing a hospital birth would relate to medical issues that your partner may have such as heart disease, kidney disease, tuberculosis, high blood pressure, obesity, serious anemia, epilepsy -- if her previous births were stillborn, breech or if there was premature labor before the 37th week. Other reasons would include toxemia, baby too big for her pelvis, problems with the RH compatibility. These reasons would all be understood before the birth, and would help you settle on making an informed choice.

However, you have other options these days. Going into the hospital can mean giving your autonomy away. Hospitals have all sorts of procedures that have become standardized and may be a big interference in the way you and your partner may want the birth to go. Many hospitals control whether you partner will have an episiotomy, be placed under the electronic fetal monitor, or have her bottom shaved. They may stop a woman from giving birth in a position she desires, routinely break the waters and perform inductions. They may cesarean 50 percent or more of their births (in 2002 the overall rate was 26.1% nationally – the rate was only 5% in 1970). Also the hospital may control who can attend the birth to the point of eliminating your partner's friends and family.

If you find you desire a hospital birth or have to have one by default, you may want to ask a whole lot of questions as to what rights and choices are available. This is the best way for you to protect this experience.

Home Birth

The opposite end of the spectrum is the option of having your baby in your home. This is obviously the least restrictive environment, but one where higher risk pregnancies can become problematic. Obviously, this option is only for those without medical complications. Studies have shown that having a baby at home is the most satisfying experience for women. In the United States, midwives are generally the practitioners willing or able to assist at these births. Often these births are not covered by insurance.

Those in the medical community usually believe that birthing at home is highly dangerous though in hospitals statistically more women and babies die (four to five times as many per thousand). Doctors have told women who chose this route that they are taking their lives as well as their unborn children's lives into their hands – this is a scare tactic. This negative attitude has existed for a hundred years and is part of the legacy of birth in American – *see Chapter 9 -- The History of Birth*. When serious complications do occur with a birth at home, babies and mothers as transferred to hospitals (the average rate is 8%). However, some people feel so strongly about birth, that they disregard the law. To them it is a political choice.

Many states require midwives to have state licensing, but some states still abide by archaic laws thus making midwifery and home birth illegal. However, ACOG wants to eliminate this option altogether. They have joined up with the AMA to issue policy statements that will threaten to make home birth illegal. Not all doctors are in support of this ridiculous idea.

Birth Centers

Instead of delivering in a hospital, some choose to use a birth center. Usually the center is staffed with midwives. The costs are generally lower than with a hospital, but few of these centers exist nationally. The National Association of Childbearing Centers reported in 1994 that 140 centers were in existence and 60 were in development. These centers are usually well connected to the medical establishment and transfer to a hospital in case of an emergency is easy to arrange. Currently, the American Association of Birth Center (www.birthcenters.org) lists about 195 accredited centers in the U. S.

Alternatives

In some hospitals there are alternatives to choose from. Some have maternity clinics that employ Certified Nurse Midwives (CNMs). Because direct entry midwifery has been illegal for so long, many women with a passion for birth, went through the specialized training offered in nurse-midwifery programs. Generally this option is covered by insurance and provides much less interventions. The safety records of birth centers and delivery by midwives in the hospital are superb.

Many hospitals have tried to improve upon having their births in the ordinary antiseptic hospital rooms; they have prepared rooms that look more like a home environment. The rooms are very popular. Yet, the veneer is all that. Don't expect the cosmetics to make the birth more in your control. You are still in the hospital after all, and the policies and procedures don't shift with a pretty set of curtains or linens.

Overall selecting the right environment is the biggest factor in the outcome of the birth. You get what you pay for and if you want control over the environment to protect your loved ones, then sometimes it makes sense to pay for expert help in an environment you want. Many people just go the cheap route by using their insurance and have a hospital birth where the hospital controls everything. That doesn't need to happen. You have rights when you enter a hospital (See Appendix C: *Patient's Bill of Rights*). Learn them if you are going into that environment. Remember when you are in the hospital, it is like you are renting that space – you and your insurance company. They are service providers and you have the right to make decisions on how care is administered. Not everyone in the hospital is going to force their procedures on you. If the nurses are telling each other how to protect patients from unnecessary interventions for their birthing mothers, then you need to understand that you better be able to advocate for your partner. So if you have the cash available and midwives are legal in your area and accessible, think about paying for the alternative environment.

Choosing the Players

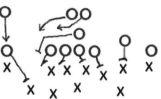

If birth were a sport, think of what would happen if in a team sport, you lost control of who was allowed into the playing field. What if the fans step out into the scrimmage or what if the coach was replaced during the middle of the game? Chaos would ensue. All sense of decorum would be lost. That is why the selection of players who come into the environment is critical.

As part of your birth plan, your partner should identify the type of people you want to involve in a birth. Some women go to the hospital without any supportive relatives and friends. Can you imagine? Why should this happen? On the other hand, you may need to size up if even her friends and relatives will be supportive. We all have seen family who will step into a situation and impose their *superior wisdom* and knowledge into whatever the circumstance. They are kings and queens yielding power. For sanity's sake screen them out of a birth. Don't let you partner be beaten into submission by strong willed family or friends. This is critical – if they agree with her birth philosophy, then their help is positive. But know that not all family members will be on your team. Don't make a mistake and not screen out the naysayers and the negative thinkers. Look at your birth philosophy and screen out those who will threaten the very environment you are creating. It's like having the enemy inside the camp.

Choosing the players also includes choosing the professionals who assist you with the birth. You and your partner may pick someone out of the yellow pages to handle your birth. You may have a choice of two doctors from the HMO. There are only so many midwives in your locale. You have doctors, certified nurse midwives, obstetrical nurses, direct entry midwives, certified professional midwives, Doulas, birth assistants, yourself and your partner.

So choosing a birth team of people with similar birth philosophies is critical. It's like getting everyone on the same frequency. Everyone needs to speak the same philosophical language at the birth. Ask plenty of questions when interviewing potential care providers to facilitate understanding.

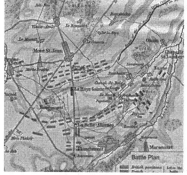

If you give up your choice of who can attend the birth, you may let others dictate the tone of the birth environment. When you cannot bring in her family and friends, don't expect to have a home-like birth. The rules are for the work environment, to make it work for them not you. Try to learn what the rules are for any location you and your partner are considering.

Ask a lot of questions. Learn what percentage of births are surgically delivered by the practitioner you are evaluating. Also know what rates the facility you are looking into have as well. If the information is withheld, you need to know why. Shouldn't you be given the odds? Also the more resistance they show in providing this information, the more you know they will resist your plans for a natural child birth, if that is your choice. You are entitled to this factual data. Be persistent. The medical profession is supposed to let you know the chances of a positive outcome. Many people do not understand the significance that a traumatic cesarean has on women. A cesarean birth needs to be treated with the same respect as vaginal birth, and it needs to be recognized that in addition to it being a birth it also is major abdominal surgery. A woman is not only depleted from the experience but has a long road to recovery which requires much more delicate handling and care.

Furthermore, inquire about the costs associated with the birth. Ask "what ifs." Are they making a medical or an economic decision? Hopefully in this book, the data here will open your eyes to the realities of what you can expect.

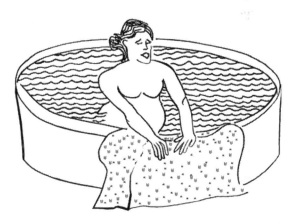

Also know what freedoms your care providers will have at the birth. Can you go to the hospital with a non-hospital-paid Doula? Who do they allow your partner to bring with her? Know what the midwives can do or not do because of the environment. These questions of protocol and policy are dependent upon what environment you are in. If you and your partner choose to birth in a tub, where can you do that? If your partner wants to walk around during labor, can she do that? If she wants to position herself in an odd way, is it allowed? Is she given freedom, or is she under someone's thumb?

Tactical Choices

Just as each armed force of our nation has different strategies and styles in their work to protect the country, each couple will have their own style in the way they would like the birth to go. These differences are highlighted in an array of birth techniques.

The first style we like to call the medical/technological style. Many people choose to have their babies in the hospital because they have an affinity for medical technology. The electronic fetal monitor is just such a piece of technology. Men especially like learning about the printed data on the paper strips being spit out of the machine. It's like science fiction. The machine monitors the contractions, their length, their strength, the heart rate of the mother and child, etc. Some people sign up (elect) for surgery, whether it is necessary or not. They think of birth as a medical event not as a natural event. You may feel more comfortable with that and so may your partner.

A second style is called the Leboyer philosophy and is based on Dr. Frederick Leboyer's book <u>Birth without Violence</u>. He states that a newborn baby is extremely sensitive to the emotions surrounding it – anger, anxiety, fear, impatience or calm, serenity, etc. He believes that the stimulation to the child should be kept to a minimum, with low lighting, few sounds, little handing and immersion in water at the baby's body temperature. Very few hospitals allow the pure Leboyer method, but will allow Leboyer-based birth.

A third style is the Odent type. This doctor preferred to allow his birthing mothers to have complete freedom to act as she wished, encouraging women to reach a new level of animal consciousness. He believes that high levels of endorphins, or nature's painkiller, should be allowed to be stimulated in the mother's body during labor. At his clinic mothers move into any position they desire. She can sit, walk, stand, eat, drink or do anything. Women seem to change positions at different times during labor even squatting to use the force of gravity. Dr. Odent is quite happy to birth a baby in a tub of water as well.

Yoga adherents may use a method based on this ancient exercise/meditation philosophy. Those using yogic methods believe women can best handle the pain of labor through yoga control. Like mind over matter, they believe pain can be controlled. The idea is controlling one's awareness.

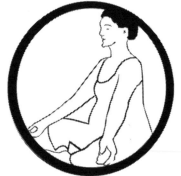

The most popular technique in the United States is the Lamaze method. This method focuses on breathing techniques as a preparation for labor. Usually this method works on developing a team, and you as a man are expected to be the breathing coach. Your job is to coax and support your partner. You must take the classes with your partner. This method reinforces the idea that the woman is responsible for her birth, and you participate with her in these exercises to prepare for the birth event.

Another doctor-developed technique came from a book titled <u>Childbirth Without Fear</u>, written by Dr. Grantly Dick-Read. This method teaches that tension and anxiety control pain and that by alleviating the mother's fear and negative emotions pain is reduced. This method also looks at breathing exercises, and includes relaxation techniques.

Another method which takes a very natural approach to childbirth is one based on Dr. Bradley's teaching. Like in Lamaze, the focus is a natural, non-interventive birth. The approach emphasizes no drugs. You as her partner are supposed to assume the role of coach. You are to be her main emotional support.

In all these methods, pain is attacked. Every couple may find themselves lining up with one or parts of some of these techniques. Books are specifically written to teach these methods, and, like Lamaze, you may find a practitioner to teach you and your partner how to use one technique. These techniques do not take away from the fact that birth is a huge emotional and physical challenge for your partner. Your participation in the planning for the birth and involving yourself in childbirth education classes or through reading will be a huge lift for her. Birth is a major trial that requires perseverance and taxes most women. Your support will help to ease this burden.

North American Obstetricians

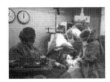The United States and Canada are two countries where the vast majority of births are in the hands of highly skilled surgeons called obstetricians. These doctors generally do not come to your partner's birth until the very end of labor (second stage). They generally show up for the delivery, all the while giving the nursing staff orders from wherever they may be. It is funny how their statistics show that most of their births are done Monday through Friday between 9 AM and 5 PM. Statistics show that emergency cesarean sections occur commonly on weekdays during the daytime. Could these doctors be requiring surgery to make birth convenient?

Why is the cesarean rate in this county higher than in other countries? In other countries midwives out number doctors and they aren't going to use interventions without cause and because they don't benefit financially if there is a surgery. The average obstetrician makes $275,000 per year. They profit by reducing the time they spend on each birth. Data from several states show that women receiving Medicaid have the lowest level of cesarean births. It is those with good private insurance who have more interventions and surgical procedures especially if they deliver in a private hospital. Doctors can make more money from the insurance where all their interventions are covered.

Another reason the obstetrician has in pushing for interventions is that they are afraid of lawsuits and having their malpractice insurance rates increase. Seventy percent of obstetricians have been taken to court (obstetricians have the highest rate of lawsuits in medicine and the highest rates of error in prescribing medications). Medical doctors routinely use an electronic fetal monitor without any medical justification. They need some tangible documentation in case they end up in court, so the machine's printout is used just for that purpose. In 2002, 88% of women were subjected to this machine – that's over 3.5 million women. Doctors may also perform a cesarean when there is little or no medical reason. The fundamental part of the Hippocratic oath is to do no harm. But, major abdominal surgery is much more dangerous than vaginal birth for low risk women. But greed and fear make a dangerous mix.

The United States has over 35,000 obstetricians and about 5,000 midwives. Great Britain has 32,000 Midwives and 1,000 Obstetricians. Britain has less than an 8% Cesarean rate and the US has more than 30%. 80 percent of births in the U.S. involve some surgical procedure; remember obstetricians are highly trained surgeons.

75% of women have a surgical procedure that cuts the vagina. This is called an episiotomy. Less than 5 to 20% should ever need this intervention – usually you are told it will stop a tear. Facts are that this operation means more bleeding, more chance of infection, more painful sexual intercourse for months after the birth, and more probability of the deformation of the vagina. Women do tear if steps aren't taken to lessen that chance. Most obstetricians just cut, taking no care to make sure the vagina remains intact.

Midwives

There are very few midwives in the US. The doctors in this country have stifled midwifery for over one hundred years. There was a concerted effort by doctors to eliminate their competition. Out of the 5,000 midwives in the country, the vast majority are nurse midwives working for doctors at hospitals. Many states still consider midwifery illegal though this may change. Some others lock midwives up for practicing medicine without a license, while other states are now establishing licensing laws.

Midwives generally have a similar belief system about birth that includes the following four points:

1. Informed Clients

Midwives believe that the more knowledgeable consumers are the better choices people will make regarding childbirth. Informed choice is stressed.

2. Family Centered

Midwives actively encourage women to involve their family and children in the birth.

3. Freedom

Midwives encourage their clients to birth their way. They encourage women to have the baby as they want. This gives a woman freedom to scream, moan, be held, walk around, listen to music or whatever seems to fit the birth mother's personality.

4. Time Intensive

Birth is time. Midwives spend as much time as is needed working with their clients. They will stay for hour upon hour until that baby is delivered.

Chapter 8: Knowing Your Enemy

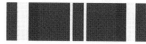

What are the Enemies of Birth?

You may not even believe any enemies exist when it comes to birth. You may have the idea that you can trust that the professionals are in control. But birth is an event of huge proportions. All that is negative and all that is destructive is the enemy of bringing a precious child into the world. You need to challenge your own fears, denial and apathy. So wake up! This is important!

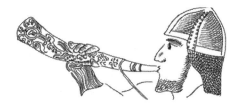

The first enemy you must confront is your own apathy and ignorance. The better trained you are and the better you know the birth mother, and understand the natural course of birth, the better choices you can help make during the pregnancy and birth. We suppose that is the way it is for everything. So be a good trooper and "Be Prepared."

The Enemy of Apathy

If you do trust others to handle everything, you may have to face the enemy of apathy. Not caring enough for this critical event in your life will leave you robbed of all its wonder and joy. Have you ever noticed that the person who has done all the reading and seen all the films, who has a real interest in the topic, is the one who is going to enjoy the experience the most? Apathy, or lack of interest, is just the opposite attitude. Whatever you focus on, and study, and prepare for is exactly what you are going to derive pleasure from.

But this is birth, and it is your mission to help provide for a safe birth. So, if you don't follow through and get involved, you may make poor choices that will have negative consequences. Remember birth is like a test. The more you know and the more you understand about its implications, the higher your score. By reading through this manual and taking childbirth education classes, you will be best prepared to derive satisfaction from the whole affair.

Did you ever have that hot car you wanted? Did you read about it? Did you check out a web site on it? Did you know how many cc's or horsepower the engine had? The more you knew, the more important the car became. Now turn that around and look at your partner. What do you know about her? What do you know about the coming child and the birth process? Most likely, half of the child's characteristics will be directly from you. The more concern and attention you spend on studying for the coming birth and the pregnancy, the more value you are saying the child and mother have in your life.

A big shame in our society is that men have participated in the take off, but will not complete the mission. That is why there are abortions. No commitment. No value. A child should have the greatest value. The fact is that our society has abandoned the value that sexual pleasure and commitment go hand in hand. So, if you want to make your own life more valuable, realize how valuable this birth experience is in not only your partner's life, but in your own.

Talk to a couple that want a child and can't have one. The barren woman has a crushed spirit. They would give anything to have a child. The cost would be their very souls we're afraid. People will go through all kind of bureaucratic hell just to adopt. Of course, if our society valued children more, there would be more children to adopt as there would be less aborted.

So your apathy shows your lack of value for the mother and coming child. Start thinking about what a child's value is to you, and then meditate on what it should be valued. For many the newborn could be the most precious thing in the world, and for most of us who have had children and held them in our arms, we realize that.

The Enemy of Ignorance

Have you ever heard anyone say, "I didn't know that was bad! If I had known, I wouldn't have done it!" Our ignorance can cause huge errors of judgment. The issue of caring is a character issue, but the issue of ignorance is one of information. Either way you go, you end up with the same result. You blow it.

So defeat the enemy of ignorance by learning. If you value this birth and pregnancy and this mother and this child, you will learn all you can about your place during this expedition. In this book we talk about birth being like flying a sortie. You need to 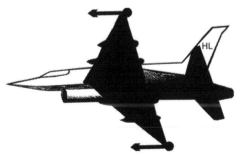 see yourself hurtling forward at Mach 1. Do you think the air force would allow a pilot to fly a multi-million dollar fighter without extensive training? Of course not! They aren't going to give that pleasure to anyone but a winner, someone who really knows his jet.

You want to take this training seriously, so that you are prepared for all the obstacles that are involved with birth. You need to know the enemies of birth. You need to plan the mission, and you need to be diligent.

The Enemy of Fear

Yes, fear is the ultimate enemy in life: Fearing the future, fearing the birth, fearing that all will go well. These fears can dominate your mind and your partner's. You need to eliminate fear from your vocabulary. You need to develop your partner's courage. That's what encouragement is all about. So eliminating fear is a huge bonus in birth. The mind focused on fear closes down that natural flow and rhythm of life and birth.

This is not the easiest of tasks, because we all feel fears. Crazy thoughts run through our minds. Capturing those thoughts and eliminating them is the overcomer's way. And, if you can handle your own uncertainty, then you will be able to stand firm and assist your partner to overcome her fears.

If you give in to fear, you become the enemy. And that is true of your partner. That is why you need to know your captain (partner). But, if you are walking around in fear, you then become the source of trouble. So know yourself as well and communicate with your partner that birth is not something you can personally handle. If your needs are addressed and you are not forced to ride out the birth, then you can be more supportive for her needs by insuring, if necessary, she has someone else who can provide the level of support needed.

Hostile Territory

As we've discussed already, the birth environment is extremely important. Eliminating the negative factors there will help the most. The fact is that once you are there, you can hardly go back. That means if you choose to have a birth at home, you have given up the support of a hospital. As a matter of fact, if you do that and try to transfer to a hospital because there is a complication involved, you should know that you will be resisted. On the other hand, if you are in the hospital and things get complicated and the heat is on, you will have a hard time getting out of the place.

We are not advocating either route, though we've been at both places. What we're saying is that you need to think things out. You need to be prepared for handling these contentious and sometimes hostile situations. The fact is that you may be being forced into a birth scenario you absolutely abhor.

Also don't forget to know the people who will be attending this birth, since they have a lot to do with the environment. The more negative the person, the more manipulative and controlling they are, the harder it will be for you to keep the environment safe and harmonious. When you hire a birth team, you should not think just because they work with birth that they are qualified. No, you need to know more about them. Mainly you need to know yourself and your partner's desires and then hire people who will accommodate those wishes. Again, the enemy of apathy and ignorance should be defeated by the confidence you have in your birth team you assemble for your birth. Yes, claim the responsibility for birth and you have made the first step in the right direction.

Negative Expectations

You should know several things about the people and the environment in which the birth will take place before you choose to let that into your mission plans. The thing to be looking out for is the expectations. If you learn that the place you are going to have a baby has a low c-section rate, you are lucky. Many North American hospitals have a 50% rate. In Europe where birth is still mainly in the hands of midwives, the rates are low like 5 to 10%. In the U.S., the midwives' rate is close to 4%. This is the expectation you should have. Like betting on a race, you should bet your money on the positive environment.

You may find that the hospital or medical practice will not release their stats on interventions and c-sections. Why should they withhold these figures? Go figure! So ask the questions: Interview staff, interview doctors. Research this before you choose your doctor or midwife – see the appendices for prewritten questioners. Get random references not just references that are sold on the service provider's work!

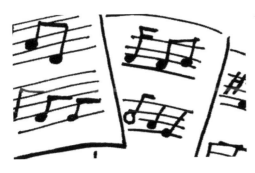

When Phil had knee surgery, he asked around for several months, trying to find someone with a great reputation for excellent results. Why shouldn't you do the same for a birth? You should have someone you trust, and whose judgment is predicable from the past. Do they have the same birth philosophy as you? Think of philosophy as a style of music. If they aren't playing your music, why would you want to dance?

The Enemy of Routine Interventions

You will find that the Medical Model is use to dispensing interventions. This model will bring an IV pole and supplies saying, "Here we go, lets' put in the IV." This is a medical intervention; the idea is that when your partner needs drugs, or replacement fluids that everything will be in place. A healthy laboring woman should be able to maintain proper hydration simply by drinking adequate fluids throughout the course of the labor. From the vantage of the Medical Model, this is what birth is like: your partner is in labor; utilize continuous electronic fetal monitoring (EFM); give all laboring women an IV just in case. The labor isn't progressing. Give the woman pit. If there is fetal distress, then prep for surgery (in some hospitals this is done when you walk in the door – shaving a woman's pubic hair and starting an IV).

What you don't know is that this stream of orders comes from the routines used in the hospital. Make sure your doctor has given the order. But if you haven't researched your doctor, he or she may be making decisions you would not approve of. You might be surprised to learn that some doctors even tell the nurses to increase the pitocin levels during inductions until there are signs of fetal distress so that the child must become an emergency cesarean. They aren't going to tell you that, and the nurses certainly are not allowed to.

Patrick Houser writes in his book <u>Fathers-To–Be Handbook</u> on page 150 the following:

> Suppose that a modern form of a father's protection is to guard against the excessive interference of people, equipment, and artificial drugs into the very ordinary process of birth. Many interventions at birth are the result of over educated professionals with good intentions who are medically trained to intervene in a non-medical process.

When you have a child in the hospital, you can do some things to keep these interventions at a minimum. It is your partner's birth, and she and you should be making these decisions. Having a Doula, a midwife or another trained birth assistant with you to fend off unnecessary routine interventions is a good thing to do. Some men take on this responsibility themselves, but most guys aren't ready for that. You can ensure that the birthing mother is continuously drinking between contractions, if pressured about IV access you can negotiate a heparin lock for quick IV access without the encumbrance of an actual IV and IV pole which inhibits her freedom of movement.

If the institution insists on the EFM, then you can agree to a short 10 -15 minute strip upon admittance to the hospital and that be all. Contractions and fetal heart rate can be measured by palpation and auscultation with a fetoscope or Doppler. The information gained by the trained ear thru a fetoscope or Doppler can be much more accurate than the EFM, and when assessing the baby's well being it seems that you would want the most thorough and accurate evaluation possible. Human touch and attentiveness is not subject to the technological glitches of doubling or halving of fetal heart rates nor is the auscultation by fetoscope diminished by the change in a mother's position as can occur with the continuous EFM. The person taking the fetal heart rate simply adapts their position to that of the laboring mother to get the baby's heart rate.

Choosing to have the baby at a birth center or another more private location just strengthens your ability to stop these interventions from starting. However, you also need to have a backup plan in case things really do have emergency written over them. If you have a midwife, you will probably have very few interventions, but you should be sure that your midwife has a transfer protocol and a proactive backup physician who can provide for a transfer to a hospital if needed and with limited conflicts.

Fear of Incompetence

The last category you should mark as your enemy is the incompetence of your care providers. Make sure that they have a track record not just a positive attitude. Though babies are delivered all over the world without a competent professional around, birth is still one of life's activities that influence a family for years. In North America, OB/GYN's have the highest number of medical malpractice cases in all of medicine. A bad experience can happen even with competent people, but you certainly need to find the best care provider possible.

Again, interview, research and record the results. Who is available for your partner's care? Be involved. Know the costs, and know what kind of practice the Doula, midwife, birth assistant, doctor, hospital or facility has. What are their stats? Ask the right questions and you'll get the answers you need to make good decisions.

Fear of Interferences

Last of the great fears are those often overlooked and that is interferences to the birthing mother. According to those involved with birth, interferences are those things that distract a woman from getting into the birth. The presence of anyone who can distract or interfere with a mother from having the birth she wants can pull her out of the focus she needs to have the baby. Birth is so intense and delicate chemically that noises and distractions all need to be removed. You see the thinking part of a woman's brain needs to shut down while the primal brain moves the birth along. Removal of chatty people, television, in-laws, and outlaws and repetitive examinations and procedures with need be eliminated. But, you may be the biggest interference. You may need to remove yourself if you are making the birthing mom unable to release into childbirth. She needs not to be talking or thinking for the birth to ease.

Chapter 9: History of Birth

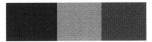

In North America

Before the 1900s, birth was considered a natural phenomenon. As medicine progressed, a new specialty called obstetrics was developed. These physicians have done everything in their power to make midwifery illegal in North America. Their motives were to improve American medical schools that were competing with European medical schools in the late 1800s. 19th century literature about obstetrics mentions how poorly trained obstetricians were and that that was due to the few hands-on experiences they had in schools. Since women did not have a right to vote, male doctors found it easy to eliminate female midwives by encouraging legislatures to adopt laws eliminating midwifery. New York State passed the first law against the practice of midwifery in 1896. By 1917, the law passed there was used verbatim to eliminate midwifery in California, so the idea had spread across the country. Only in the southern states where doctors did not want to eliminate the midwives did midwifery survive for some time – these doctors just wanted to train the midwives. Yet most doctors agreed that to improve medical schools they had to raise the standard of obstetric instruction and by eliminating the midwives they could take on more observations and hands-on training. Doctors were also very concerned that with the statistics for their profession. In the early 1900's New York City midwives delivered 40 percent of the babies and had 22% of the deaths. That means the doctors had 60% of the births and 78 percent of the deaths.

At first only wealthy women first chose to use doctors at birth as it was a sign of prestige. The idea that one has a private doctor for one's delivery became a must for upper class women. Only the poor continued using midwives, until midwives were branded as practicing medicine without a license. For years afterwards midwives were forced to work underground or to stop their practices.

As the doctors took over birth and while they harangued the midwives, birth moved from out of the home and into the hospital. In the 1940s, 44% of births occurred at home, but by the 1970s less than one percent still happened at home. Consistently, obstetricians recommend all birth to occur in the hospital, though the empirical evidence has never shown a reason for this—thus it is the doctor's bias that has changed the landscape of birth. More amazing is the fact that the populace has agreed to their dictum.

"The increasing preeminence of the physician drove the changes in the practice of birth and spelled doom for the traditional practice of midwifery. This increased involvement of doctors altered the philosophy of birth by systematically redefining pregnancy and birth as pathology that required medical treatment and encouraging childbearing women to view their condition as one demanding medical care and sure that only male medical professionals could adequately provide. This redefinition of birth advocated an increasing interventionist approach, thus altering the practice and the cultural construction of birth." Birth Chairs, Midwives, and Medicine by Banks, Amanda Carson

Since the early 1970s, the women's rights and the anti-establishment movements awoke women to rethinking their lives. Birth was part of this change in mindset. Midwives began working again even when they had to do this covertly. Hippies had their children in communes. Midwives still helped the poor women have their babies at home. But, obstetricians controlled birth, and they were at their apex of power and position. During the 70's, women were placed on tables with their legs up in stirrups. They were not allowed to have their husbands or partners with them when they delivered. Birth had become totally medical. The business of birth began to be handled like a factory – routines were devised to shuffle the populace through their doors. The doctors had created the "Birth Machine." This machine was designed like other forms of big business and industrial enterprises. The procedures and techniques employed by these doctors became used throughout North America; after all they believed in their way of handling things, for to them birth was a medical emergency.

Another source that provides a nice overview of the history of birth is at the following web address:

http://www.ourbodiesourselves.org/book/companion.asp?id=21&compID=75

Today's Doctors: Trained to Distrust

Medical schools train their students to distrust the nature of birth. The study of obstetrics focuses on the abnormal birth and the multitude of problems that can come up in a very small percentage of births. Complications in birth are what are sought out. Their textbooks are literally filled with malfunctioning birth scenarios. Little attention is ever focused on a general uncomplicated birth. Due to their training, they handle birth as if it were a heart attack or life threatening injury.

Medical school is said to be dehumanizing, a type of emotional, intellectual and physical harassment for the student. North American medical schools are highly competitive. Many of the students when asked why they want to become doctors will tell you point blank that they just want to be wealthy and that is their motivation for going through the horrendous rigors required. The amount or materials covered in these schools is immense and the amount of effort required to become a doctor is incredible. Interns are pushed to the limits as well, running 12 hour or longer shifts. This type of process reduces people and creates medical professionals whose care is brief, dehumanized, and stressful.

Where does that put the average obstetrician? No wonder why doctors spend so little time with birthing women, seen mainly as birthing machines which can break down any minute. They do not look at birth as a personal human experience. They see that women are weak, cannot have the babies on their own, and that it is their job to save the life of the babies.

Birth is their territory and will be done according to their desires. This makes it easy for them to make your partner's birth fall within their time schedules and routines. They have x number of births to do in a day, so they wait around for any signs of complications. That is what they are trained to handle. Staff are given specific parts of the birth to attend to and trained only to handle their area of expertise. Doctors rely on machines, tests and "science," rather than on the perceptions that their clients have. This is not personalized care. Your partner will find most often that she is just a number, some tests, etc. in any large medical organization.

Outside the Medical Model

As birth in North America changed, other industrialized nations did not follow course. Midwives were still practicing in Europe. By the early 1980s, after years of reduction in morbidity of women and their children, something happened -- medicine was unable to continue to improve the levels of mortality. Factors that were social in nature were frankly out of their reach. Many women who had poor diets, lived in poverty, etc. were delivering babies of low birth weight -- these births have substantially higher mortality (more babies die). The situation could not be addressed without a change in the way birth was handled. The sterile, inhumane environment of the hospital could do nothing to stop low birth weight babies. This was, and remains, a serious social problem.

Thus, many who work with birth worldwide began recognizing a second approach to birth, which is called the Social Model. Instead of looking at birth as an emergency about to happen, these professionals looked at birth in the light of anthropology, sociology, and psychology. Instead of looking at birth as an analytical medical issue, these folks looked at birth as it related to the individual and the community. Birth lost its impersonal cold face and adopted one of triumph when a woman achieves fulfillment.

Many interventions used over the years by doctors proved dangerous and were dropped years after their use saturated the industry. X-rays were done routinely on pregnant women for about thirty years until a 1956 study showed that children had an increased chance of developing cancer. Interestingly enough the mortality rates of women did little to improve once the doctor had gotten midwifery legally abolished. Then, when World War II occurred and the doctors were called out of their specialized work with birth, the mortality rates fell an unprecedented degree. But after the war, the reign of doctors and their technology continued with hospital birth becoming the standard. 44% of birth in 1940 occurred outside of hospitals, but by 1970, only 1%. Consistently, obstetricians recommend all birth to occur in the hospital, though the empirical evidence has never shown reason for this—thus it is the doctors' bias that has changed the landscape of birth.

Mythos as Fact

However, the industry that the doctors built was still hard at work, and is part and parcel of the cultural view that Americans have been brought up to trust medicine completely. People think of and speak of birth as a hospital experience. Medical-oriented birth is the standard for our culture. People believe the mythos that birth is intrinsically dangerous and that the hospital is the safest place to have a baby. The doctors' point of view has won the day.

As North Americans, we are raised to believe in machines. The industrial and scientific revolutions focus on mind over matter, science over religion, machine over nature. Technology is applauded as the salvation of all things, even combating death. Nature is seen as something to be controlled and mastered by science and technology. Birth is just another of the natural conditions that have fallen under the purview of this thinking. It's part of the culture.

The birth machine has taken birth from out of the natural process and used the higher valued science and technology over nature. One description refers to this situation and compares it to salmon spawning. In nature the fish swim up stream and leave their eggs. In our culture of machines over nature, we would handle it by damming the stream, extracting the fish by machines, force them to spawn artificially, grow the eggs in trays, then release the fish near the ocean.

After a birth, the birth machine and the technocratic philosophy continue to grind away at the natural process. Babies are taken from the mother; painful shots are administered; and they are placed in rooms with other babies where their chance of getting infectious diseases go up – all for the convenience of the hospital staff. Then even the breastfeeding time, the best time for child nurture and care, is put on a timed schedule. That is one of the main reasons there has been a movement toward attachment parenting. For the birth machine the clock has provided the main frame of reference, creating regimentation reminiscent of the factory, forcing breastfeeding into the series of steps – always focused on time and efficiency. Completely distrusted are natural signs that women and their babies have. Women have a letdown where their breasts are saying, "Hey, let me feed the baby." Then the babies are crying and saying, "Hey I'm hungry," but the birth machine says "the parents and babies need to learn discipline." But science, the supposed foundation of the doctor's world, declares that this idea has no empirical basis.

Historic Procedures

Much of the routine interventions used in hospitals came out of research done many years ago. The medical world generally follows those procedures even if they aren't scientifically relevant any longer. Though all the research shows the dangers of having a woman labor on her back, it is still being done. Though the "No Eating and No Drinking" rules came from the anesthesia dangers of the 1960's, this is still protocol. Other routines like enemas, shaving the pubic hair, taking the baby from the mother, IVs, all of these are products of historic misinformation. Modern studies repudiate these procedures.

Medical Communication

The history of medicine in the United State reveals that doctors are trained to conceal information from their patients in order to promote a position of superiority and dependency. Women's records are coded with abbreviations and medical jargon. This ability to hold the power of knowledge over a woman's head is the basis of all professional interactions. Many doctors will outright resist a woman's having her own medical records, believing that only they can make decisions related to health care. Remember this is the culture of medicine, not necessarily a conscious effort on the part of doctors to thwart communication.

Doctors have been socialized to speak in medical gibberish to mystify health. The less a woman knows the more power the medical establishment has. So your partner will want to know what is in these records and stay informed about her body and health. So if you want to improve your partner's access to information, you can demand your medical records – and wait to see what type of consternation this causes. Also you could keep your own medical records for the pregnancy. Information leads to power. When you and your partner are informed then you can choose the best options for your childbirth experience.

The decisions of the health care policy making groups are all in the hands of men though there are women in pediatrics and gynecology and obstetrics. The leadership of all international and most government policy making groups are all men. Women are dominated again. However, women are the central issue here and their reproductive rights and safety are at issue.

The routine hospitalization of pregnant women is widely practiced regardless of the scientific evidence of efficacy and the hardship this places the family. This hospitalization is expensive and disruptive. Usually people don't know they have the option of going home. They just do whatever their doctor orders. This is the culture of North Americans. Yet if everyone has recuperated from the birth, why stay. You might not be surprised that hospitalization is recommended even when there is not medical justification since your insurance covers it.

History of Abuse

In the past the birth machine used a drug called scopolamine, a drug that wiped out the memory of the birth and labor. The women were actually awake but like wild animals. Many had to be tied down using lamb's wool to hide any marks. "Doctors and nurses, looking at such behavior induced by the drug they had administered, felt justified in treating the women as crazy wild animals to be tied, ordered, slapped, yelled at, gagged (Harrison 1982:87—Harrison, Mitchell 1982 A Woman in Residence. New York: Random House)." This type of abuse isn't so prevalent today, but many women find themselves chastised and belittled for questioning the current common procedures, recommended by the birth machine.

Measuring Outcomes

If the efficacy of a measure or technology has been demonstrated – that is, if the methods of prevention and intervention that are of interest have been shown to work, we can then turn to measuring the effectiveness. But in the case of ultrasound, when the efficacy has not been proven, then you cannot look at effectiveness or efficiency.

In the birth industry, the technologies used may not have efficacy, but they are employed. Ultrasound as a case in point is used regardless of its efficacy. The instrument has taken the place of a trained pair of hands in measuring the growth of the fetus. Doctors only spend ten minutes at an appointment. They send women to ultrasound so they won't have to spend the time to do the measurements – even when accuracy is compromised.

This type of care is not sensitive and not supportive. It is sterile and dislocated. The doctors aren't even using good science. They offer a risk approach to birth. That means they run tests to see if your partner is at risk. The more risk generated the more involved the obstetrician will be. Your partner becomes a passive patient who is given little choice. The risk approach makes pregnancy an unnatural thing. The pinnacle of this approach is the high-tech hospital. Saving lives is the idea, but the whole approach is focused on the negative – about what can go wrong, and with the lousy accuracy of some of the testing, these tests just increase the stress and anxiety of women. Since there have never been scientific definitions of normal, obstetrics treats all birth as risky.

One of the central problems in the system is the scoring of what constitutes high risk. Data is taken from women all the time to determine their risk level – as a score is then assigned. Every epidemiologist knows that using 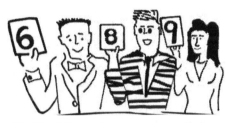 population statistics to apply to an individual is a dangerous technique. Scales have been developed, but their efficacy for the prevention of morbidity and mortality has not been clearly shown (Marsden p. 99). Those placed in the low risk category still have complications, showing the inaccuracy of these scoring mechanisms, and it also means that those in the high risk category who have all the extra testing – which can be very dangerous, never needed those tests. Furthermore, this can erode a woman's confidence in her ability to birth naturally. This risk approach is the current perspective of birth in the vast majority of hospitals in North America, but worldwide the approach fails since it is unable to predict the risks well.

The Role of Men

Historically, women birthed in a room with other women: sisters, mothers, aunts, grandmothers and their midwives. Men heard birth, but they were not overly involved. They were still connected, because the births were happening in the next room. Many people outside of North

America still see birth in this universal way. Birth is part of their lives; they remember births of their siblings and they still think of birth as a womanly art. When medicine took birth away from the midwives, this shifted the place men had in birth. The sterile environs of the hospital replaced the bedroom. Birth was cordoned off and men were totally separated.

In the 1950s and 60s, when the hospitals began giving women that drug that made them like animals, men were never allowed in labor and delivery rooms. The medical staff didn't want them to see their women behaving so badly, so men were locked out. Believe it or not women demanded the right to use this procedure, just like women demand to have their cesareans and epidurals today. Men had no idea what their women were going through, and we suspect they would have raised hell if they had only known.

After the Cultural Revolution of the 60's, the men in society were adjusting their thinking. It wasn't just a sexual revolution that occurred, but it was a mindset, expanding and rejecting the norms of the day. Men started demanding to be involved in birth. As these attitudes changed, and as medicine itself changed, men began attending births. Then in the 70's they began coaching birth through the Lamaze and Bradley methods. They participated and they made their presence felt. But for some men, they still didn't want to leave the waiting room. They would rather not know what was happening. They felt out of place and awkward.

Over time, at the majority of births, men accompanied their partners into the hospital, hoping for the best, trusting the machine to deliver to them a healthy mother and baby. They signed the consent forms; they blindly accepted the dictates of their doctors. They said yes to drugs, surgeries and to timetables. They also learned to sue doctors if anything really bad happened. They gave up their authority over birth, knowing that their insurance would pay for nearly everything. It was the North American way. Everything was going to be all right – the doctor was there! And if not they had an attorney.

As birth became more and more interfered with, some couples went to birth to fight off the interventions. They became a team to protect birth. Others decided to have their babies out of the hospital and at home. These folks began bringing in their friends and family and even their children. Birth bounced back into the public eye so to speak.

These changes have had a rippling effect in North American society. The vast majority of women still birth in the hospital today, but men are now accompanying their partners. This is considered normal now. No more are men sitting in the waiting room ready to hand out cigars. Even cigars are not the gift of choice.

Are Men Causing Trouble When in Attendance?

Now we know many birth philosophies exist that include men at the birth, and this is a result of the swing back of pendulum. Once men were removed from childbirth, they now are often center stage. But not all men are cut out to be at the entire birth scene and this can negatively affect childbirth, so we thought we should say something about that.

Dr. Odent, a famous obstetrician who has attended 15,000 births, has recently stated a new interesting position about the place of men at childbirth, and it is something we think is worth considering. Dr. Odent discusses how men can become stresses and release adrenaline in the birth environment which causes women to become stressed, thereby lengthening labors. The idea is to remove all stress from the birthroom. The article may be referenced on Daily Mail at the following site:

http://www.dailymail.co.uk/femail/article-559913

Dr. Odent brings out a lot of points that are counter culture to the 70s trend of having men as labor support at births. Other points to ponder from this article relate to whether all men are positively affected by their childbirth experiences. The emotional impact according to Dr. Odent can cause men depression or cause relationship breakups, if they are not able to handle or process the strong emotional experience.

Another major point is whether men's presence actually brings the calm and peace necessary for the woman to relax at the birth. If conflict or stress results, then it is best for men to be out of sight, and we can concur as this was our experience. That is why it may be more effective for men to make it their mission to protect the birth environment and pay for proper birth support rather than take on the emotional weight that childbirth involves. So it is best, most likely, if you can't handle this strain to take a secondary role. Women need for their bodies to birth to be able to enter another mind set where they are not thinking and certainly not stressing. If you attend the birth, then you need to be calm, collected and never distracting. You do not have to attend a birth to accomplish your mission, but you might actually negatively affect the birth by being in the birthing room. However, the key is making the environment a place where she can be totally secure and able to birth. Remember the polar bear hunts down all enemies of cub-birth and eliminates them.

History is Being Made

Who can say what has been lost or gained by the way things have developed in the U.S. One belief is that birth should be part of all of our lives. It should be as much a part of life that we appreciate the intensity of the experience and the joy of a successful landing. We should know the sacredness of life and the solemnity of death. Honoring our partners by celebrating birth with them is an event we shall never forget. Instead of talking about the touchdown pass at the end of the super bowl, or the grand slam that won the series, we should one day tell our sons with much pride how their mothers triumphed in childbirth.

Whether you attend the birth or not, by being involved with your child's birth shows you are giving your best. We want you to know that you and other men are writing a new chapter in the history of American childbirth. You can help change how birth is handled, where birth takes place, and who are the professionals involved. Once men are no longer ignorant about these topics, then they can help to create public health policy, and be more understanding and supportive of women's needs.

Chapter 10: Safety in Childbirth

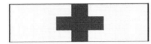

Facts and Fiction

One thing you should know about the birth industry is that a lot of money is at stake. One fifth of all medical revenues are generated through maternity wards, because of birth. Like any other profitable business, medicine is going to sell you their services. They especially quote and believe "birth is the safest in the hospital." But that isn't true. Scientific papers have shown the safety of out-of-hospital births and that "normal infants fared worse in larger hospitals."

It is important to remember that it has never been scientifically proven that the hospital is a safer place than the home for a woman who has had an uncomplicated pregnancy to have her baby. Studies of planned home birth in developed countries with women who have had uncomplicated pregnancies have shown morbidity and mortality rates for mother and baby equal to or better than hospital birth statistics for women with uncomplicated pregnancies. These studies have also found significantly fewer interventions used in home births than in hospital births.

Obfuscation

Recently two major medical studies were done which when reported were twisted to deceive the public. The first was a comparison of home births to childbirth in the hospital. This study took place in Washington State and, of course, showed that home birth was dangerous compared to hospital birth. The doctor had eliminated from his findings all the births in the hospital that required medical interventions such as cesareans, forceps, vacuum extraction, etc. so that doesn't exactly compare apples to apples. This doctor's intent was to mislead the public. He has a very good reason since the facts show that more mother and infant deaths occur in hospitals, besides all the other traumas and injuries received there.

Another study was done on the probability of rupture of the uterus in vaginal births after previous cesareans. The study showed that a very low probability exists for rupture of the uterus unless the woman had already had a cesarean. Yet it neglected to describe that the chance of rupture was equal to those without the surgery unless the doctor used induction drugs like pitocin and others. So what is interesting is that the American

College of Obstetricians and Gynecologists (ACOG) then demanded that women with previous cesareans be forced to only have their births in hospitals where they can be monitored. This type of twisting of the truth really shows that the populace is feed lies. Medicine is supposed to use science and logic to write health care directives, but clearly that is not the case in obstetrics which is not using evidence based care.

So what are the facts about safety? Wouldn't you like to know?

Measuring Safety in Childbirth

When you compare birth in a hospital to birth in freestanding birth centers and home births, you shouldn't be surprised to find that birth is always safer out of the hands of the surgeons. If you chose to have your baby in a hospital, you run greater risks. A birth in a hospital generates the following multiplications of risk (Rothman 1982:44):

- 5 times maternal high blood pressure in the hospital
- 3.5 times meconium staining (indicative of fetal distress)
- 8 times shoulder dystocia (shoulders stuck after head is birthed)
- 3 times the rate of postpartum maternal hemorrhage
- 3 to 7 times the need to resuscitate baby
- 4 times the babies become infected with diseases usually bacterial
- 30 times the babies suffered injuries usually from forceps

> injuries include blood beneath the scalp causing anemia
> fractured skull
> fractured clavicle
> facial nerve paralysis
> brachial nerve injury
> eye injury

- 9 times more severe tears of the perineum for mothers
- 9 times more episiotomies (cutting the perineum)
- 5 times more cesareans

Practitioners from the technological model of birth will use all their medical skills and knowledge to keep the "dangerous situation" from killing both mother and child. They believe they are there to save life and limb, but this approach causes a huge amount of negative outcomes. These procedures are inherently risky and often cause injuries as noted above. The birth machine is not gentle. When women birth at home with other women, their chances of having a gentler birth are high. Birth in the machine is physically, psychologically and fundamentally hard.

Perinatal deaths are higher for doctors in hospitals than for births in the home. This news has been around for some time, but the medical community has wanted to suppress it or to manipulate the statistics to skew the figures. In one study the rate was 18.1 per thousand deaths for doctors in the hospital and 2.1 percent for midwives in the hospital. Midwives delivering at home had one death per thousand at home. In another study, the stats for homebirth looked worse than those of the hospital. The caveat was that the figures for home births included non-planned, emergency home births, where women were birthing quickly and not planning to stay home. The rate was 17 per thousand in that study, but eliminating the unplanned (and unassisted) home births, the rate was 4 per thousand, when the hospital was 16 per thousand – this study was done in 1974 in North Carolina.

What is taking place in the United States and Canada is quite different than what happens in Europe. Historically these other nations still use midwives. In Europe, 75% of births are attended by midwives (from Health Watch, Nov 1997, Vol. 2 Issue 7, p. 4). Medicine in North America is supposedly the best in the world, but the US has a relatively high mortality rate for babies, ranking 28st among major developed nations. Why is that? Two factors contribute to the poor showing of North American obstetrics. First, unlike Europe where women are supported by social programs, North Americans have little governmental support. What is more obvious is that the majority of births are handled by male doctors and surgeons rather than female midwives. The very technologies used by the birth machine are eliminating the human touch.

Safety with Midwives

Comparing births in hospitals to birth with midwives is a difficult task, for midwives screen the births they take, ensuring they have few high-risk pregnancies. Generally besides having better mortality statistics, they provide a much gentler and humane touch to birth. As mentioned before, midwives average 1 hour per prenatal meeting with their clients, while doctors spend on average 10 minutes. Midwives (which means "with woman") basically stay the entire labor with their clients, rather than showing up for the last 30 minutes, as is the case with many obstetricians.

Ina May Gaskins, a famous midwife from Tennessee, reported that out of 1707 births she attended 95.6 percent successfully delivered vaginally. 4.4% transferred to a hospital. None of her mothers died and eight babies died (3 from lethal birth defects, 1 from respiratory failure, three from severe prematurity, and one of unknown causes). The neonatal mortality rate was 4 per thousand. These statistics are comparable with other midwives.

Beyond the fact that less women and babies die, midwives handle birth with an alternative philosophy. They don't look at birth as a medical emergency, but work with their clients to engender a supportive harmonious environment. They also do less damage to the babies as shown above where interventions cause physical harm.

Similar statistics show up with freestanding birth centers. Out of nearly 12,000 births at freestanding birth centers studied in 1989, the overall cesarean rate of 4.4% and the perinatal death rate was 1.3 per thousand.

What Causes Babies to Die?

Each year, 35,000 infants die in the U.S. before their first birthday.

> 20.9 percent of birth defects
>
> 16.6 percent from prematurity
>
> 14.1 percent due to Sudden Infant Death Syndrome
>
> 4.6 percent from complications of pregnancy
>
> 2.4 percent from accidental injuries

Add to that that the miscarriage rate is 31%. That's huge. That means 3 out of every ten pregnancies end this way. Women for whatever reason can lose a baby quite easily. This is a common experience for women.

Most babies who die have neurological problems that inhibit the baby's being able to live or they have undeveloped principal organs like kidneys. Prematurity is the second main reason -- low birth weight of babies is the most common factor in perinatal death and in neurodevelopmental handicaps. It is hard to pinpoint the cause of these defects, but nutrition is a fundamental to proper growth and maturation.

Most surprising is the Sudden Infant Death Syndrome stats. All of our children were raised with the attachment parenting philosophy. We like keeping the baby in bed with us. It made nursing more convenient when our daughter who was premature by one month and Genny was recuperating from a cesarean section, so we adopted it. We had read about it one of Dr. William Sears books, and thought it would be nice to try. Once our youngest son was only a few weeks old, he stopped breathing in the wee hours on the morning. Genny noticed that he had stopped breathing, and reached over to him and pulled him to her bosom. This stirred him, and he began breathing again, but it gave us quite a shock. You can't be awake for every minute of your baby's first year, so it paid off having him so close by.

Social Interventions

Many social factors like poverty, domestic violence, inadequate housing, poor diet, stressful life events, lack of social support, smoking and the abuse of alcohol and drugs have a harmful effect on pregnancy and birth. These factors often can contribute to low birth rate, which is the most commonly associated phenomenon. To counter these negative social factors, social interventions are used. Most importantly, the developing baby needs to have a good environment in which to grow. Social interventions help women get off drugs, stop smoking, eat nutritional foods, exercise and be removed from dangerous and/or abusive living arrangements. Most of the socialized countries of Europe have programs like these in place, but they are sorely lacking in the United States.

A social intervention program that can make a significant difference in the health of newborns is changing women's smoking habits. Studies show that women who smoke 20 cigarettes per day during pregnancy have a 60% chance of delivering before the 33rd week. Women who continue smoking have a 25% greater risk of fetal and infant mortality. It makes sense that preventing premature babies would improve the health of newborns and should be a priority of North American healthcare, but, unfortunately, according to studies, 30% of clinic patients who smoke don't even hear the mention of their stopping smoking from the clinics they visit. This social intervention is not valued as it ought to be.

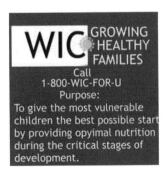

Nutrition during pregnancy is another major social factor. One study showed that women who participated in the WIC (Women, Infants and Children) were matched against women not participating, and the WIC pregnancies had lower incidence of low birth weight, lower neonatal mortality and increased gestational age. This means fewer babies died and they were born more mature and healthy. Medical intervention for improving the safety of birth are not addressing these social issues, and it is plain to see that improving a woman's diet and reducing her negative health habits do make a measurable difference in the birth process.

North American medicine needs to be reformed so that these social interventions – the prevention method of healthcare – are adopted. The perfect example of how wrong things have gone is in the case of what happened in Indianapolis, Indiana. People in this city learned that their city's infant mortality rate was the worse in the country for large-sized cities. The folks studying this from the medical community suggested that an expensive, high-tech medical van be purchased and sent into the poor neighborhoods. The machine was equipped with the latest ultrasound equipment. This, of course, did nothing to improve the lives of the poor pregnant women in the city and only proved to be good for the companies selling the high-tech solution. If they had only stopped and spent the money of distributing high nutrition-packed foodstuffs, then they could have made the difference. Taking a truckload of peanut butter, eggs, high quality whole grain bread, and cans of tuna to distribute through the neighborhoods would have done more good. Instead the $1,000,000 medical van was driven into poor neighborhoods, causing no improvement in the statistics.

Sadly, it is reported that poor women are clearly worse off than women who are incarcerated in federal, state, and county jails where they receive a regulated meal plan and better quality food.

We heard an interesting story about a young American service man living in Ireland – his wife had just had his baby girl in the Irish hospital. When the Irish nurse came to discharge them, she brought vouchers for butter, cheese, milk, juice, and other foods. The guy kept trying to refuse these, saying he was an American and that he didn't need the help. But the nurse pressed the vouchers into the wife's hands, saying to him, "You may be an American, but this young lass is Irish and she is entitled to everything the Irish government wants to give her.

Who is in Control?

Of all the major institutions in our country, only government and the military are as authoritarian as medicine. Prenatal care through the medical model almost always encourages compliance with medical advice at its core. The ideology is to assure that women comply with their doctors. The focus is the convenience of the medical staff. When doctors control birth, we already see that risk increases, with 4 times as many deaths.

When birth is shifted out of the hospital, these risks are reduced mainly because interventions are not used to hurry the birth process. Both home birth with midwives and births in freestanding birth centers give the control of the birth to the woman. Hospitals trying to improve their image and to provide a more home-like environment have set up alternative birthing rooms in suites in the hospital. These rooms look very nice, having pretty curtains, a nice bed, and a separate bath, but they are births still controlled by modern medicine. 40% of first-time mothers actually deliver in those rooms, the other 60% end up down the hall in the traditional labor and delivery rooms. You have to be kidding yourself to think a birthing room in a hospital is any different than the regular hospital despite the cosmetic wrapper. The power of the birth machine controls the whole scenario. As one doctor put it, "You are still on the doctor's turf and you will play by the doctor's rules."

Mother Safety

Fortunately, throughout the industrialized world, medicine has reduced much of the risks to mothers. Long ago, many women died due to hemorrhaging or from getting infections. Antibiotics took care of much of this problem, along with the development of blood transfusions and other modern treatments for blood loss. Women still face risks. This is especially true of those having significant interventions like a cesarean section.

In the United States, 31 out of 100,000 women die of this surgical procedure. Compare that to other risks. 26 out of 100,000 women die from breast cancer, 20 out of 100,000 die from car accidents. 6 women out of 100,000 die during spontaneous births, so your partner has 5 times a greater chance of dying during surgery. Out of all the midwives we've read about, none have had a woman in their care die. It is with the surgeries where the risk of death to your partner goes up. Think of it, your partner has more chance of dying from a cesarean than from having a car accident or from breast cancer.

The medical model is not readily going to tell you the serious risks involved with the procedures they use; however, using inducers, giving a woman drugs, getting an injection in the spinal cord (with epidurals), having major surgery (as with a cesarean section), all these procedures can cause significant problems and lead to death. Especially dangerous is giving a woman who already had a cesarean section inducers which can hyperstimulate the uterus and cause it to rupture as mentioned above. Induction drugs are dangerous in and of themselves, so why should they be used at all? It has to do with controlling the birth with any available means. You see they don't want to wait; they want to be in control. Few practitioners from the technological model will sit and wait for the normal physiological order of birth, nor would they trust a woman's body to handle the process without their interventions. This is the key point. The birth machine thinks that a woman's body is like a mechanism, and if it isn't performing fast enough they infuse and inject it with chemicals to get it up to snuff. It doesn't perceive the intuitive nature of childbirth.

VBAC

ACOG has ruled that trials of labor for women attempting a vaginal birth after cesarean section (VBAC) must be run only in the hospital. This governing body exerts a great deal of political, social and legal power in the United States. Their rule also forces doctors to have to be in the hospital during the whole course of the labor. What doctor can do that? None. The bad news is that until this ruling is lifted, most midwives will not take on one of these "high risk" births. Actually a multitude of excellent studies document that a vaginal birth after a cesarean section is not a high-risk pregnancy. What makes it a high risk is the procedures used by obstetricians.

If midwives were to take these births, then they could lose their licenses. Even women who have had several successful VBACs, like Genny, would still be considered "high risk." It is funny how the whole thing is controlled by the medical establishment. They control what is considered high risk. They control how a high-risk birth is to be managed, and they eliminate the option of a lower risk birth environment. This should not be.

If your partner is thinking about having a VBAC, then until this ruling is overturned, it feels and appears that the birth machine has all the cards. It is critical to the success of a VBAC to have the support of your birth team. Achieving a VBAC is not impossible; the statistics for subsequent pregnancies resulting in a vaginal delivery should be equivalent to that of women who have never experienced a cesarean. Ideally a woman should anticipate she has a four to six chance out of a hundred to require a repeat cesarean. With the accommodating health care practitioner, and supportive birth environment one should be able to deliver vaginally. Your search for a supportive and accommodating birth practitioner may be difficult, but continue persevering if a VBAC is what you both want. Birth is significant. Empower yourselves with Nancy Wainer Cohen and Lois J. Estner's book Silent Knife: Cesarean Prevention and Vaginal Birth after Cesarean (VBAC), also Cohen's Open Season: A Survival Guide for Natural Childbirth and VBAC, and take advantage of the resources available through International Cesarean Awareness Network (ICAN), www.ican-online.org. Genny found these books and this organization to be invaluable in working through our traumatic c/sec birth experience and in equipping us to see our dreams realized with subsequent vaginal births. We cannot underscore the importance that a woman with a previous c/sec deserves to be treated equitably, and in just the same manner as a woman who has not experienced a surgical birth. Remember uteri without surgical incisions rupture too. The medical establishment's premise that a VBAC is a high risk birth is that once the uterus receives an incision then it is more likely to rupture in subsequent births, however uteri that have never been incised have ruptured during birth also.

The Objective

The ultimate objective for any birth encounter is a good outcome for both mother and baby. A successful birth experience no matter what the outcome will be one that enhances the longevity of the family. We have outlined the safety risks for you and your partner to be aware of. What is really great to know is that eating right, proper exercise, and a lifestyle free from cigarettes, alcohol and other drugs can greatly improve a woman's chances of having a healthy baby. You can play a big role in helping your partner achieve these things. Yet, on the other hand, if you chose to be lackadaisical about the forthcoming birth, and resign all responsibility of the birth to the birth machine you encounter higher risks for negative outcomes. By paying particular attention to the desires and needs of your partner, you as a couple choose the environment for having your child. If she gives birth in a hospital, you must remain cognizant of what is done there, or better yet secure the services of a Doula who understands and can advocate for your birth philosophy for you and your partner. The birth belongs to you and your mate; it is fitting that the decisions to be made, that you have control of, be made by the both of you. It is easy to be intimidated by the austere environment of a hospital; however, a consumer needs to understand that they are paying for the services, and they have every right to determine what happens in the space they are paying for.

Chapter 11: Quality Healthcare

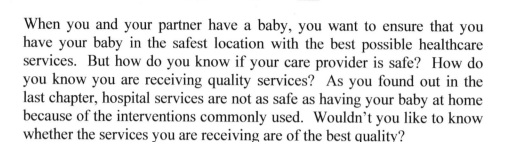

When you and your partner have a baby, you want to ensure that you have your baby in the safest location with the best possible healthcare services. But how do you know if your care provider is safe? How do you know you are receiving quality services? As you found out in the last chapter, hospital services are not as safe as having your baby at home because of the interventions commonly used. Wouldn't you like to know whether the services you are receiving are of the best quality?

Measuring Quality in Services

The three "E's" of measuring quality in health care services are Efficacy, Effectiveness and Efficiency. To understand how health care quality works you need to understand these three terms.

First, the least familiar term is Efficacy. This means that a technique, procedure, drug or treatment has proven successful in controlled research. This is how medicine is supposed to work. A new treatment is investigated and it is documented by comparing a control group with another group. These studies take a lot of time and effort.

Effectiveness is about its use in real life. If a treatment works in a controlled experiment, such as the testing of a new drug, than it may have high efficacy, but if no one will take the medication because it tastes awful, then it has little effectiveness. So assuring what treatments are effective does not mean they work, but rather that they are something people will receive. So when a treatment proves effective, that doesn't mean it works, but rather that it is well received.

Efficiency is the evaluation of the cost benefit ratio. Is this method affordable? If the drug we discussed is effective, and it is affordable, than it is efficient (Epidemiology by Leon Gordis, p. 45). So when you have a high cost solution that is paid for under insurance, medicine can offer that to you instead of a cheaper solution. That is inefficient. But when something cheaper is used instead, such as using the generic, that would be efficient.

How do these terms play into the subject of birth? First of all, many of the techniques used by modern obstetrics have not been thoroughly tested for efficacy. The technique may be effective and bring about the results the physician wants, but that doesn't mean the safety of the technique has been evaluated in clinical research.

Since medicine has a heavy bias for implementing costly technological interventions in birth, they often chose expensive technologies over labor-intensive approaches to solving birth outcome problems. This is extremely inefficient. Rarely are random controlled trials of birth technology done because of these biases. HMO's have learned how effective and efficient midwives are and have turned more and more to using them for their hospitals.

Birth Machine Techniques: Safe or Convenient?

Many people want to have their baby where the best of modern medical technology is available. They trust that this technology has been effectively tested and that the practices of the doctors and hospitals are based on scientifically based research. That is not the way it is. Let's look at some of these techniques and discuss how these techniques affect childbirth.

Enema and Shaving

Enema and shaving are still used in hospitals though these practices are unnecessary, and historically are done before abdominal surgery. Both have been cited as ways to reduce contamination, but studies have proven this false. So why keep up a practice of this in the hospitals? Neither technique is scientifically necessary. Women are still constantly asked if they have eaten and given an enema, which is painful, to make sure there is no food in the woman's system. Physiologically this is crazy. The woman needs energy to birth. The purpose is to prepare the patient for anesthesia if surgery is necessary. Take the energy away and you are bound to increase the chance of surgery because your partner can easily become fatigued. Try running or just walking 15 hours on an empty stomach. So both practices are designed for the convenience of the hospital. Women do not want either of these done to them. Psychologically such procedures reflect a woman's giving up of her autonomy and accepting the sterile environs of the medical world. Women are often very compliant with any medical requests, so someone needs to make sure these intrusions are avoided. Stay off the procedural conveyor belt of the birth machine and refuse to have the enema and the pubic shave.

IV Therapy

Why an IV? Many hospitals prohibit laboring women from having fluids, just in case they have to do a surgery later with anesthesia. If your partner has fluids and then surgery, you are told she can throw up and asphyxiate. The birth machine is designed on the medical model, so the norm is that IVs are used throughout the hospital, especially for giving drugs intravenously; however, medical research shows that IVs are not a harmless way of providing fluids to a woman's body. Complications from IV therapy such as infiltration, where a catheter goes into the surrounding tissue and the IV fluid enters tissue instead of the vein, or hematomas, where the catheter punctures the vein and blood seeps out into the tissue forming a pool of blood, are not unheard of.

This practice of not giving fluids orally to a person in surgery came about during the 1940's when anesthesia was administered through a mask. So it made sense then, but today, intubation is used, placing a tube down the throat, so no food or liquids makes no difference. Only 2.6 persons die from asphyxiation out of a million and mainly because the person giving the anesthesia was incompetent.

This practice has denied laboring woman food and drink during birth. Midwives never deny a woman food and drink. People believe incorrectly that IVs are harmless, so they accept this old standard practice. Dehydration and starvation negatively affect both your laboring partner and the baby, both of which need plenty of energy and liquids. Any of us who are athletes understand that at strenuous stamina-demanding events one needs to eat carbohydrates before the activity and get fluids during the event to perform effectively – the same is true of a birthing woman. We tell guys that labor is like lifting two dumbbells of 25 pounds each for one minute with a two-minute break between reps. The catch is that you have to do that for 12 hours without eating, though you may have ice chips. No one we know of will try that, but you get the point. None of us would starve ourselves during an athletic competition of endurance.

Starving your partner can lengthen her labor, wear her down, and give practitioners cause to use pitocin, which can make labor harder to bear, etc. Feed your partner. Give her fluids. There are some excellent sports drinks that are high in calories. There is a drink called Ultrafuel™. It has like 120 calories per 8 ounces – perfect for extremely demanding sporting events. Remember there is no reason when you walk in a hospital to have an IV when you are pregnant. The IV is for the administration of drugs. The IV is for the convenience of the staff.

If you can't go without, a good compromise is to request a heparin lock, which allows for an IV to be added easily by the medical personnel. It allows them to have quick access to drug administration, and your mate the ability to move around without the encumbrance of an IV pole.

Why Cervical Checks and Vaginal Exams?

Cervical checks are routinely done on women. These can be painful, lead to infection and basically have no medical need behind them. Why are women subjected to these? The focus of birth in hospitals is providing that a woman is proceeding with her birth. The measurements used to determine that are based on averages for all women. Any woman taking a long time to birth is suspect, but all women have their cervix routinely checked. The information obtained from this procedure is very superficial and inaccurate. The risks are that the gloved hands transfer germs inside the cervix. The birth canal is covered in bacteria, so by sticking anything up through it to the cervix, increases the chance of infection for the birthing mother and her baby.

The point of the vaginal exam has nothing to do with safety; it has to do with seeing how far your partner has advanced in labor. However a vaginal exam is only one way of assessing a labors progress -- as the midwives say, you know a woman is coming along by the flow of birth fluids and mucus. You don't need to see the cervix's size to know when it is time to push, the woman knows instinctively – unless she has been drugged.

More Serious Interventions

Amniotomy

Amniotomy is the surgical procedure for breaking of the bag of waters. This procedure can reduce time of the first stage of labor by about an hour. In two-thirds of women, this bag of waters does not break until the second stage of labor. So an amniotomy is an artificial maneuver that can just disturb the physiological timing of the spontaneous rupture. Though it may be of benefit to the doctor by reducing the time of labor there is no evidence that it is of benefit to the mother or baby. Actually once the waters are removed, trauma to the baby's head may increase, causing swelling to the skin of the baby's head, misalignment of the cranial bone, and possible higher incidence of fetal distress. When the umbilical cord is tampered with and compressed, this means that the blood supply to the baby can be interfered with, upsetting the delicate chemical balance.

Research has shown that amniotomy produces a reduction of maternal uterine blood flow of sufficient length to lead to metabolic and respiratory acidosis (Wagner 1994). More significant is the loss of the protection to the umbilical cord, which can now be compressed during contractions – the bag of waters is a natural cushion that prevents this. If the umbilical cord comes out before the baby, a prolapsed umbilical cord occurs. One now has a situation of great danger to the baby where the baby justifiably will need to be delivered immediately.

Scientific studies have never shown that amniotomy is healthy, so as with any other intervention offered to you consider why the procedure is being presented and whether or not you and your partner feel that the benefits of the procedure outweigh the risks. The only time it works well is when her cervix is all ready prepped and softened up. The procedure fails often since most hospitals have the twenty-four hour rule – this means the baby is going to be born in 24 hours or else. The fear is that infection can result just as in the rupture's occurring naturally. But clinical studies show that the infections have more to do with the frequency of vaginal exams – the bringing of a foreign object into the birth canal.

Rupture of Membranes

The medical world makes a big huge deal about when a woman has her bag of waters break. The ruptured membranes can reseal. A tremendous concern exists that among other things infection may set in. Infections can occur especially if people are continually examining the cervix. A woman may simply monitor her temperature over the course of several days to insure the evaluation for possible infection. She also may wear a sanitary napkin to assess whether or not any fluids are continuing to leak. Labor does not necessarily immediately proceed after the membranes rupture, and unless infection is suspected, there is no need to have surgery or to be coerced into a labor induction. After a rupture of membranes has occurred and all is stable with no evidence of a prolapsed cord or other complication, there is no reason why a mother cannot monitor herself for signs of infection by taking her temperature twice daily and adhere to other precautions regarding sexual activities. Obstetrics means to sit and wait and the words of one of Genny's favorite obstetricians rings true; "As long as both the mother and baby are alright do nothing and watch and wait, if and when either the mother or baby demonstrate they are not ok, then and only then do you intervene. So as long as mother and baby are doing fine leave it alone.

Remember if you arrive at the hospital because her water broke, and she is just starting labor, you have just given yourself over to the dictates of the birth machine. You can monitor the signs for infection and the early labor yourself. It is not a good idea to be afraid of anything, and since the bags of water break early in about one third of women, this is very common. In 8 – 10% of term pregnancies membranes will rupture prior to the onset of contractions, according to studies, but 60 to 95% will start labor spontaneously after the water breaks without further intervention. By keeping probes and hands out of your partner's vagina after her waters break you are doing everything possible to avoid infections. But when the bag of waters is broken unnaturally, a woman may not be ready at all to have her baby. Failure to progress is a main reason hospitals write down for their reason to do a cesarean section.

Induction

Here is a common chosen procedure that the medical model offers. Either starting a birth with drugs or hastening a woman in labor is induction. Many of the procedures we have covered are clumped together with induction – one intervention leads to another! This procedure is the real sign as to how invasive medicine has gotten in birth. Generally this is all about making birth convenient for the physicians, hospital staff and even for impatient mothers. By trying to speed up the process through drugs and other physical factors, more babies could be born between the hours of 9 to 5 when the doctors are in the hospital. Many studies have proven that this is the current case in North America. In some ways it has become a choice that is offered by physicians to women since many women desire control over when they give birth. Anyone knows when they are around a pregnant woman that when she hits that last month, she can't wait to have her baby – for many it is as if they were saying, "Get the kid out of me." Induction seems to be the choice.

Induction starts now with a chemical(s) being administered to bring about contractions. Usually pitocin, a synthesized version of oxytocin, is administered via an intravenous drip. The benefits are for those women who face conditions like pre-eclampsia or the psychological issues related to carrying a stillborn. Anyone can see that hurrying up labor is beneficial in those situations. It is an entirely different matter to consider induction for post-dates that is when a woman goes past her due date without going into labor. The mantra from that astute Midwestern obstetrician, "As long as the baby is doing well and the mother is doing well then leave it alone" surfaces hear as well. It is wise to consider that during the last weeks of pregnancy the fetal brain is developing at rapid rates and to deliver before the baby is ready may very well mean robbing him or her from additional brain cells.

The risks of an induction are more pain in labor since the intensity of contractions heightens. Induction can cause uterine hyperstimulation that may in turn lead to inadequate placental blood flow oxygenation and fetal compromise. This means that the baby's blood doesn't get the oxygen and this endangers the baby. The stronger contractions can also lead to fetal distress.

Once an induction is initiated, you may find further complications developing. It's like taking the stairs. You find that the induction drugs wear a woman out, causing fatigue and pain. This may lead to the use of drugs to cut the pain since "pitocin often causes uterine contractions to be more intense and painful," or to possibly sedate the woman. Often labor ceases and there is no more progress – since exhaustion can occur. Those hazards are so clear that another technology is introduced to monitor the progress of labor. Yes, instead of sitting with the woman, that medical world created an electronic fetal monitor, with readout and everything. This robotic sensor takes the place of constant nursing care.

The natural replacement of the drug induction of labor is to have your partner walking around and using nipple stimulation to speed up the labor. Studies have shown that a woman's walking and moving around decreases the need for pain killers by two thirds. Another study showed that ambulation (movement) is more effective than oxytocin (pitocin) in restoring normal progress of labor. In women who have prolonged labor, breast stimulation was shown to be as effective as drugs, but caused fewer complications.

Trends are for more and more women to choose induction, but the FDA usually has restricted the use of the drugs for induction unless there is a medically documented need. The doctors get around these rules by rupturing the membranes (breaking the bag of waters). This then, according to hospital rules, requires only 24 hours before possible infection that gives them cause to give women inducers. Estimates of 75% of all births are reported to be moving to this practice. Because women want to have the baby out, they sometimes schedule a time to be induced. Two main problems exist with that: First, the baby's brain is laying down new brain cells every hour in the last weeks of gestation; and second, the woman's cervix may not be prepared properly for a birth. So choosing to have the baby earlier is a choice that can limit that positive development and growth of your child, and an induction without the cervix prepared often leads to a cesarean section.

Rupturing the membranes reduces the natural cushion for the baby's head. The sack of waters really improves the ability for a woman to birth her baby naturally and with less stress to the baby's head and shoulders, so unnaturally rupturing the membranes is another negative and unnecessary intervention. Regularly, induction follows the rupturing of the membranes. Serious problems can result if the umbilical cord descends, causing it to be squeezed during contractions – this can again cut off life-giving oxygen to the baby.

64% of women who have inductions chose epidurals to regulate their pain. Could it be that the inductions actual push the level of birth pain higher? "The prevailing norm in obstetrical practice is that the elimination of pain is a primary factor in providing a positive childbirth experience. However, effective pain relief does not ensure a satisfactory birth experience for women. In one study, mothers reported that attention, sympathy, reassurance and support were superior to epidural anesthesia for a rewarding outcome.

Many physicians today are using a new powerful drug called "cytotec" for inducing labor. This drug was designed to help stop stomach cramps. The medication is labeled with a warning not to be used with pregnant women. However, doctors discovered this drug could induce labor as it causes severe uterine contractions. A doctor wrote that it turns a woman's cervix to "mushie." The fact that the drug is being used by ob/gyns to start labor is frankly scary. If birth management followed a scientifically researched course, would these methods of induction be used? The reality is that methods such as these are hazardous. They increase the mortality rates for women birthing (Maternal Confidence for Labor and the Use of Epidural Anesthesia, International Journal of Childbirth Education, Fall 97, Vol. 12 Issue 3, p34, 5p, by Dana Stern). Some women die when their uterus ruptures, causing profound bleeding – a higher incidence of rupture occurs when the woman has had a previous baby surgically. So if these drugs promote higher mortality rates then why are they used?

The last word on induction has to do with the willingness for doctors to ignore scientific data on the techniques used. Induction should only be done in certain situations, but it is now commonplace. The medical literature, including obstetrics textbooks, describes this clearly. In the fifth edition of Human Labor & Birth by Harry Oxorn, the author states on page 688-689:

> "Before inducing labor of using a modality to prime or ripen a cervix, one must differentiate between a cervix that is unprepared and one that is already ripe….As long as the prerequisites are observed, the rate of successful labor inductions is over 90 percent."

A test called the Bishop's score is taken to measure this. The book further states on page 689:

> "When a high score is present it can be assumed that cervical ripening has taken place and no further attempts to ripen the cervix are needed. According to the Bishop's system, the

maximum total score is 13. When the score is 9 or more induction of labor is always successful. When the score is four or less, failure of induction is common and pre-induction cervical priming should be performed."

POINTS

	0	1	2	3
Dilation of cervix in cm.	0	1-2	3-4	5-6
Effacement of cervix (%)	0-30	40-50	60-70	80
Consistency of cervix	Firm	Medium	Soft	
Position of cervix in the vagina	Posterior	Mid	Anterior	

What is obvious is that you do not want to let your partner be induced if her Bishop score is lower than 9, and you must resist adamantly if the score is 4 or lower. It is reported that doctors will (1) break a woman's membrane (rupture the bag of water), to get the first stage going faster, then (2) will administer pitocin, and (3) then because the cervix isn't ripe, the labor will stress the baby, so (4) c-section!

Birth Position

Throughout history women birthed babies in positions excluding lying on their backs. However, obstetricians changed all that. These doctors were trained to do surgery on people lying on their backs. So naturally the stirrups on beds were created to suit the doctors' convenience. It is easy to do a vaginal examination when the woman is on her back.

Studies show that being on the back is the worst position for bringing forth the child. Women who were in a vertical position during the first stage of labor were found to have 25% less time to advance than those on their backs; for women having their first baby, this difference was 35%.

Studies show that when women are given the choice they prefer to be seated, walking and standing (and having the choice to change position) during the first stage of the labor. They prefer the squatting position during second stage contractions, while seated in between those contractions. In these studies women never chose the "on your back" approach.

Logically, you face more resistance in birth from having to drive the baby horizontally than vertically. Gravity is a force here that should be used. A hospital bed is usually considered no comfort unless it manipulates into a chair form. Birth chairs have been used for centuries (all the way back to the Pharaohs of Egypt). Babies born to women using such a chair are shown to be healthier due to lower rates of fetal hypoxia (oxygen deprivation).

Several studies show that using the "on your back" position causes the uterus to compress the main blood artery from the mother's heart to the baby. Contractions are also weakened by the position, which slows labor. Pushing during the second phase of labor is strongest when a woman squats, less strong when she sits and weakest when she lies down. So having your partner lying down has both a negative effect on the mother and the baby and it can compromise the efficiency of the contractions.

Fortunately in North America, medicine has allowed women to make position choices. Birth chairs are a kind of compromise allowing women to adjust their position at will and allowing their care providers. Inexpensive beanbag type cushions have been employed and studied and their use significantly shorten second stages of labor and significantly lower forceps deliveries. Some hospitals actually have purchased expensive birthing chairs – since they are marketed within the normal medical profession, but an inexpensive chair is just as good.

Drugs: The Most Common Intervention

Birth is unrelenting work. It can be unbearable, especially when a woman becomes exhausted. When a woman becomes exhausted it becomes more difficult for her to stay on top of the pain she experiences. Modern medicine believes all pain should be eliminated. 77 percent of women take painkillers of some sort in childbirth. We all feel awkward when someone else is agonizing. Much of what childbirth professionals do is to help manage these feelings. "As birth is a physiological process, there is no justifiable reason for the routine administration of medication during labor or birth" (Marsden Wager, 1991), but in American society, drugs are the panacea for any medical problem.

Three types of medications are commonly given: pain relievers, anxiety suppressants and anesthesia. They all reduce the pain to some extent, but not without hazards. Both pain killers (analgesics) and anxiety suppressants (tranquillizers) act on the central nervous system and affect the respiration of both mother and baby. A drugged partner may mean one who is not fully and actively participating in the birth process. She may not be capable of psychological interactions with you and others at the birth.

Drugs taken to cut the pain of childbirth are taken into an infant's system within seconds. The baby's brain can be affected negatively, depressing its ability to resist hypoxia – lack of oxygen – and causes variability of the baby's heart rate. Babies who have been drugged score lower on the Agpar due to flaccid muscle tone, poor reflexes and inadequate or no breathing. The lack of oxygen and breathing requires birth attendants to revive the baby. Plus after the baby is born, your partner may experience pharmacological depression; this interferes with bonding and breastfeeding.

Furthermore studies have connected babies who have been drugged to have increased chances of developing serious drug additions later in life, according to the article 'Opiate addiction in adult offspring through possible imprinting after obstetrical treatment' (Jacobson et al. 1988). Despite these warnings, few women are able to avoid these drugs. It is easier for the medical staff to manage a sedated patient.

Although narcotics are available in most North American hospitals, research shows that they are not very effective in relieving pain and have risks for mothers and babies. Although nitrous oxide is not widely available in the U.S., the best available research suggests that it can provide helpful pain relief, with fewer unintended effects than either epidurals or narcotics.

It is an astounding thing to observe a baby that has just been born, that has not been exposed to drugs. The baby when placed on the mother's abdomen can locate the mother's breasts by itself. The baby in fact makes its way to the breast and begins nursing. Unfortunately with the wide spread use of pain relievers in labor suites this phenomenon is rarely witnessed in hospitals, the baby is just too groggy.

Alternative Pain Management

There are alternatives to the management of the intense sensations of labor and pain other than drugs. The alternative methods of pain relief come with no risks to the mothers and to the babies. The process of labor it self releases painkillers, as labor progresses, the body starts releasing painkillers called beta-endorphins – similar to morphine, but lacking all the negative side effects.

Human touch by a family member or a birth attendant helps to reduce pain. Also there are methods like massage, hypnosis, application of hot or cold compresses, acupuncture, etc. Water is a significant pain reliever itself. One method of utilizing water is to labor or birth in a large tub of warm water; this is known as the midwife's epidural. Genny labored and gave birth in a tub of water with one of our children and said it definitely worked for her. Genny adds, "there is something about the property of water and being buoyant that diminishes the intensity of labor; I have found with myself as well as with the many women I have attended in childbirth that being submerged in water enables the woman to relax and allow the water to absorb the intensity of labor." Women are actually able to float through a contraction. Soaking in a warm tub of water can be a diagnostic tool also especially in determining if a woman is in active labor or not. If a woman is in actual labor being submerged in water will speed up the labor, and if she is not in labor it will slow the labor down. So if there is any doubt as to whether labor is active or not, when a woman takes a warm bath and gets out of the tub and is able to go back to bed she should, but if she gets out of the tub and labor intensifies you have a good indication that she is in labor. When considering using a warm tub of water for pain relief, or to simply help a woman relax consider the fact that if a woman is less than 5 cms dilated that the effect of the warm water will slow dilatation but if she is 5 cms dilated or more the warm water will increase the rate of cervical dilatation.

What is an Epidural?

An epidural is a method of blocking pain by an injection in the spine. As of 1992, after twenty years of using this technique, it had not been adequately studied as to its effectiveness and efficacy. Studies do show how it compares to other drugs, but not much has been done to research this highly used form of pain numbing. The research shows that its use does lead to higher levels of surgical intervention. Even the risks that arise have been understudied. Your partner's short-term health issues would include possible drop in blood pressure and fever. The drug can also effect the predisposition to malrotation of the descending baby and cause the mother severe headache. In Kannan's reported study, "Maternal satisfaction and pain control in women electing natural childbirth," that for women that planned natural childbirth who during the course of labor decided to have an epidural that despite it's lowering the intensity of pain, 88% reported being less satisfied with their childbirth experience than those who did not use epidural. Studies relating to long-term health issues show women have one or more of the following: severe headaches, severe back aches, bladder problems, tingling, numbness and sensory confusion.

Most drugs are not allowed on the market if they endanger patients at a rate of 1 to 30,000. In one study epidurals were shown to have a 1 in 14,000 danger of killing birthing mothers and a 1 to 5,000 range for causing serious complications. The biggest danger is of lowering the blood pressure. Complications in mothers include cardiac arrest, respiratory paralysis (which means the mother can't breathe), allergic shock, and maternal nerve damage. Therefore the scientific studies show that there are inherent risks of using epidurals:

Loss of consciousness 1 per 3,000

Cardiac arrest 1 per 3,000

Severe hypotension (low blood pressure) 1 per 2,000

Severe headache 1 per 2,000

The babies are affected by the epidurals adversely in that often they have less blood flow from the placenta. They too have absorbed some of this drug. Common complications include the following: Oxygen deprivation, slowing of heart rate, increase in blood acidity, and poor muscle tone. Babies' Apgar scores are almost always lowered.

The main indicators for problems related to this procedure are that it leads to further complications. Common complications from epidurals include the following:

(a) prolonged second stage of labor

(b) bed confinement (sitting or laying down)

(c) loss of feeling of control in the birth process

(d) need for electronic fetal monitoring

(e) increased probability of assisted deliveries

This information was taken from the International Journal of Childbirth Education, Fall 97, Vol. 12 Issue 3, p34, 5p, Author Dana Stern, Maternal Confidence for Labor and the Use of Epidural Anesthesia.

The medical profession calls this treatment safe, though no medical literature has proven this.

Description of an epidural:

A local anesthetic is injected into the lumbar region of a woman's back, right between the ligaments and the vertebrae. Epidural reduces your partner's ability to push, obstructs with the baby's descent, and interferes with the natural rotation of the baby. Because of these factors, the probability of the use of forceps or cesarean section rises dramatically. The pain killing success is marked below:

85% free of pain

12% partial

3% no relief

Epidurals are commonly used, and so many women can tell you about their experiences first hand. Often women who have had epidurals in a previous birth will avoid them in future births. They usually complain about how the epidurals slowed down the transition point of the birth. One woman wrote "In my first birth experience they gave me the epidural when I was ready to push. I then had the baby eight hours later. The next time, I was determined to wait so they couldn't do that. I left home at 4:30 pm and had the baby at 6 pm." Other women believe that an epidural helped them relax to get through their birth experience. Some women think that the "pain free" way is the only way.

The Birth Machine's Birth Machine: EFM

Interventions like we have discussed tend to continue to be used regardless as to whether or not they have been shown to be positive for the laboring woman and her child. The EFM or electronic fetal monitor is a classic case of technology gone awry. It was first used on women in the high-risk category, but today it is used routinely for women who are low risk. This machine is designed to follow the woman's progress in labor. A handy-dandy readout strip is continuously burping forth a stats sheet for the nurses and doctors to read. The problem is that this machine has never been scientifically proven to reduce infant mortality. The machine has been said to prevent brain damage to babies, but scientific studies show there is no improvement. The idea is to avoid cp and brain damage, but studies show that auscultation (taking the fetal heart rates manually – with a Doppler, fetal scope or stethoscope) done every fifteen minutes is a superior way of monitoring for fetal distress. The EFM is cumbersome and restricts a laboring woman's movements. Women often speak of being tethered to the device. The continuous read out is designed to track the Fetal Heart Rate (FHR); however, this technology is known to interpret the maternal heart rate as being the FHR and is well known to double or halve the actual heart rate of the baby. An individual trained to take fetal heart tones can provide more accurate assessment of fetal wellbeing. An individual also can flex with the laboring mother to accommodate her positions while taking fetal heart tones. It is by far the best method; however it requires more intensive nursing care than utilizing the EFM.

No scientific evidence exists that fewer babies die if the EFM is used on all women during childbirth. Because most of this equipment requires less connection with professional support like a nurse, nurse-midwife or doctor, and because your partner will most likely have to labor in the worst position, and unable to ambulate, the machine is a big problem. Remember the best position in first stage is standing and walking, and in the second stage is squatting. Many women who birthed in a hospital and were tied up to these machines hate them. They feel like they are specimens. Hospitals love them because they can staff one nurse to watch four machines. Often health care providers just check the readout at nurse's station and leave you and your partner alone.

Medical personnel may tell you that this machine helps to reduce the rates of cerebral palsy, but clinical tests show that when comparing children monitored by the machine versus auscultation that the incidence of cerebral palsy was 20% in the EFM group while the auscultation group had rates of 8% -- this study was of children born prematurely. Children who are premature have had less time to develop their brains – might this not be a big factor in the rates of neurological problems? "The fact that the cerebral palsy rates have remained the same for the past thirty years in spite of widespread EFM is further evidence of the lack of efficacy of EFM to reduce neurological sequelae" (Wagner, p 160).

It has been said the cesarean rates tripled after the introduction of this machine. The high false positive readings from these machines place a lot of women unnecessarily on the birth machine's surgical conveyer belt. This is explained away by medical staff, insisting that their interventions save large numbers of babies from brain damage. These beliefs are based on incorrect thinking and are not scientific (Simpkin 1986). Some suggest that the machines are used to protect doctors from lawsuits – that in court doctors are able to convince jurors that the use of the monitor prevents death and/or disability? However, that may be easy to claim, but the scientific data does not prove that claim.

Episiotomy

According to medical research the cutting of the perineum is appropriate in less than 20% of women. The birth machine uses it in 75% or more. Obstetricians claim that they cut this tissue to prevent gross tears (3rd degree or worse). Scientific studies show that the severe tear rates are much higher in women who have this surgical procedure. They also show that doctors with the highest episiotomy rates are the ones who end up with a disproportionate rate of severe tears. This means the surgery actually does not prevent these tears, but actually worsens the tears. The doctors with the least amount of episiotomies had the least amount of severe tears. Therefore the claims that this operation is beneficial are clearly distorted. It is a hallmark of midwifery care for the midwife to patiently wait and to apply oil and warm compresses to the perineum as it properly stretches to accommodate for the birth of the baby. It is helpful to grasp the full measure of the subject of the stretching of the perineum when considering the web of flesh between one's thumb and finger. Our flesh can stretch to assist us in carrying a large load. The webbing may at times stretch to the point of small tears, in order to grasp a parcel. However, if you were to slice that webbing between the thumb and fingers and then try and lift the same load, you would lose the integrity of that flesh and subject yourself to a larger and greater degree of tear upon lifting that same load. It is further akin to making a snip in a piece of cloth and then ripping it. Once the snip is made the cloth has lost its integrity and is easier to tear apart.

The risks of cutting a woman's bottom include additional blood loss, elevated chance of infection – remember what bodily fluids flow and ooze from the area north and south of the cut. There is often a poor job of sewing the tissue back together – which by the way are scientifically proven to heal more poorly that a level one or two tear.

The long-term aggravations are moderate to severe pain in 60% of women. This affects women sexually. Two thirds of women who have episiotomies complain of discomfort and pain (after the wound heals of course) when they have sexual intercourse. Women report feeling sexually assaulted and traumatized – as the procedure can mutilate the female genital.

What can be done to avoid tears and surgical procedure? Well, health care professions, including those doctors with the lowest levels of episiotomies, take the time to prepare these tissues. Compresses and massage are the most common means of preparing the area for the baby's head to come forth. But the birth machine doesn't have time to address such an insignificant part of birth. The conveyor belt just runs your partner to the quick slice of the scalpel. That takes about 2 seconds, when it might take half an hour to do the massage with oils.

Cesarean Section

A cesarean section is the surgical delivery of the baby, where the baby is delivered through the abdomen while the mother is anesthetized.

There is among some obstetricians a thought process that a section is preferable to a vaginal birth. The physician cites his control of the timing and the events of the delivery when it is a planned section. Birth becomes a controlled and managed procedure, like an appendectomy. The patient arrives at a scheduled time, one that is mutually convenient for both physician and the family, for an orchestrated series of events or procedures and protocols. Looking at birth from merely the stand point of managing an event a planned section does appear appealing. However this vantage point does not take into account many serious issues. The fact is that a section is major abdominal surgery with a longer and more painful recovery time which is more susceptible, when compared to vaginal birth, to the complications of infection and death.

This surgery has many drawbacks for women and babies. The ideology that a section is preferable to a vaginal birth does not take under consideration the affect that a section without the process of labor has on the infant. The classic story of the butterfly coming out of the cocoon is analogous here. It is common knowledge that for the health and well being of the butterfly one should not intervene with the natural process of the butterfly emerging from the cocoon. The butterfly needs to strengthen its wings by the process of emerging from the cocoon and when others break the cocoon for the butterfly, rather than wait and let the butterfly emerge in its own timing the butterfly is rendered weak and cannot fly and survive. Evidence exists that a similar phenomena exists for babies during the labor process. It seems that the process of labor prepares the baby to be prepared for the birth and life outside of its mother, most notably in the stimulation of the lungs and also by increased levels of stress hormones. Labor contractions stimulate the lungs to prepare the baby for breathing and expel from the lungs the absorbed amniotic fluid avoiding wet lung syndrome. Furthermore, as the fetal head is compressed during pushing, stress hormones are released to prepare the baby for life outside of the womb, enabling the baby to be more alert which helps to initiate breastfeeding after birth.

If a child has to be delivered through surgery, the baby's health is greatly improved if it has experienced some labor. Hales 1993 illustrates "The neonates delivered by cesarean section without labor demonstrated a higher frequency of respiratory morbidity compared to those delivered by cesarean section after labor (12.4% versus 5.6%)." Women therefore who have gone through labor only to necessitate a section should feel positive about providing their child with the preparatory experience that the process of labor offered their child.

Genny adds that from a sociological perspective birth is an inherent life event for women. No one understands what the value of the process of giving birth can mean to a woman. She suspects that the process of labor and birth provides women with the opportunity to gain significant tools to cope and get through difficult times that may be called upon at later stages of a woman's life. If she does not experience childbirth and gain these skills it may place her at a decidedly disadvantage to cope with further life events. By electing a scheduled section for no other reason other than a specific medical reason she may be robbing herself of the opportunity to acquire inherent skills.

We believe that with all the benefits that labor offers to the mother and baby, and all the risks posed to the mother and baby from abdominal surgery that any so called benefit of convenience for scheduling an elective cesarean resoundingly are not worth it.

For certain complications in pregnancy and birth, surgery is a real life saving technique. Our first child was delivered by cesarean section. Women who have premature separation of their placenta, or preclampsia, placenta praevia, or a congenitally small pelvic outlet should have this procedure. For other conditions like fetal distress or failure to progress after a long and difficult labor, a c-section can be beneficial. However a review of literature about birth reveals that this surgical procedure is used well beyond any legitimate reasons. World Health Organization recommends an optimal cesarean section rate of 5% to 10% for the best outcomes for mothers and babies, and that a rate above 15% seems to do more harm than good (Althabe 2006). The cesarean section rate in the United States was 31.8% reported by the National Center for Health Statistics U.S. Department of Health and Human Services based upon preliminary data for 2007. A rate of 31.8% is more than double what the World Health Organization states as being a cesarean rate that does more harm than good. Clearly something has gone wrong in childbirth in America.

Breech births and births after a previous c-section are routinely surgical, though scientific evidence shows that both types of births can safely occur vaginally. The term used for those birthing vaginally after a previous cesarean is called VBAC (vaginal birth after cesarean). Many doctors are not supportive of VBACs and persuade their patients to undergo a repeat c-section, yet the medical scientific research proves that VBACs are still safe. The use of drugs for inductions is truly what is problematic for VBACs.

Research shows that women at private hospitals with private insurance have the highest levels of this surgical procedure. Could it be that it is opted for because it paid for? "In the United States the profit motive explained hospital specific cesarean rates that were high even by United States standards. The results were consistent with those reported by other investigators. In the United States many private health insurance packages reimburse physicians and hospitals by the procedure rendered. Therefore, more tests and procedures per patient means more income for the physician and greater revenue for the hospital" (Stephenson 1972).

Doctors also perform cesarean sections because they are afraid of being sued. Diagnostic evidence (such as taken from the fallible EFM) showing fetal distress may be enough for many physicians to perform this surgery. "Even when the diagnosis is clear, obstetricians have recently tended routinely to perform cesarean section to respond to conditions for which the evidence does not support its usefulness" (Wagner 1994).

The last non-medical reason for this serious surgical procedure is convenience. As studies have shown, inducing a woman's labor only reduces labor by an hour. So choosing a surgical birth can make birth even more convenient for the doctor. Many women who are having their first child will never make it to a vaginal birth because it takes a longer process for labor to become active than what is routinely construed to be normal to the birth machine. The concept of what is normal for length of labor has gone from 36 hours in the 1950s, to 24 hours in the 1960s, to 12 hours in 1972. Remember the dictate that as long as the mother is ok and the baby is ok then do not intervene. The criteria for what is presumed normal for a length of labor is illogical and has no scientific basis.

If you take your partner who is having her first birth to the hospital early on, such that labor has just begun, you could be in the hospital for several days. Doctors are generally not going to want to wait this out. If there is any failure to progress, then generally they are going to start intervening, though they may have no medical reason. If your partner waits however, until she is headed toward the second stage of labor, then she is more likely to be able to deliver vaginally in the hospital. So mothers birthing for the first time have a higher cesarean rate than those who are having their second child.

Level of Care

Most men have no idea how to evaluate the level of care provided for their partner. We aren't really informed about this issue. Since the mainstream is use to the level of care in the hospital, we have nothing to compare that experience with. But a few of us have gone through different types of services and we have an eye on this issue.

If you birth in the hospital the level of care will vary greatly. Primarily, your physician is not going to sit through the birth with you and your partner. They are going to rely on others to keep track of the labor. They facilitate a birth, but they are not there physically. Some doctors have even further distanced themselves from the birthing woman that they buy a computer/multimedia system that allows them to stay in touch with the birthing mother while still being in their office. They report that their patients like this because it is better than their not being there at all.

The point is that birthing with a doctor is not a high level of care. The doctor is going to spend the least amount of time with your partner. He or she may not even show up until the last minute for the birth. If there is a conflict in their schedule, you may never see your doctor at the birth at all. Frankly doctors write that they can't understand why midwives are so totally inefficient with their time.

Midwives unlike the doctors generally sit through the labor process. Even in hospitals, the midwives are going to be there much more than the doctors. It is the EFM along with differing members from the nursing staff that are going to be with you and your partner. Depending on how busy the maternity ward is, you may see little or a lot of these folks. If there are a dozen other women birthing over the same time period, the nursing staff is going to focus on who is getting to second phase.

If you birth at home or a birth center, the amount of care and attention your partner is going to receive is maximized. Midwives are going to be there the whole time of active labor. They may go in and out of the room, but they are there the whole time period. If the birth is an extended amount of time, they may take breaks for food and a catnap, but they will have an assistant who will be with you.

So the level of care is part of the quality of birth. You might compare having a baby in the hospital like driving up to the drive-through at McDonalds. The clerk is going to check your order, and then they are busy with all the other customers. The chef (doctor) has precooked the food, and only shows up to see that you are enjoying it. As the level of care rises, so does the type of service. With a midwife, you could say the level of care is like having the chef sitting at your table, serving you your wine, and having conversation with you as she cooks your partner's individually designed course.

Chapter 12: Birth Philosophies

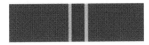

Basically two distinct philosophical views of birth exist, and you need to become aware of which one you are influenced by. The first is that birth is a dangerous medical emergency. You might call this the medical model. These people believe that they need every modern medical service available at the hospital. The other major philosophy is called the holistic model. These people believe that birth is a natural bodily process. They generally avoid the medical model. At the extreme of each philosophy are those who birth at home (holistic) without professional help and those who schedule their cesarean section (medical) regardless of medical necessity.

Birth as a Medical Emergency

The medical model basically focuses on birth as a problem, as an emergency about to happen. Women are seen as imperfect birthing mechanisms, and technology is created to repair the machinery of birth. Drugs are used to kill pain. Machines are used to record contractions. Tests are run to verify that all the chemistry is right. Doctors use their wizardry to start and stop labor. They don't need a woman to birth the baby. They can take it out quickly, if allowed, with the scalpel.

Medical papers have been written recommending cesareans for all. The assumption is that everything that can go wrong will go wrong and that every effort should be made to fix the woman and save the baby. Doctors could do this. They are trained to do these surgeries, and though the surgery is serious for the patient, it is a controlled procedure. The unknown of birth is eliminated, and that makes medicine very much in control. Birth becomes a sane predictable experience – for the doctors. That kind of thinking equates the woman giving birth like a car careening out of control coming down the raceway. Surgery just puts that car on the flatbed tow truck and delivers it to the finish line "without a scratch." Neither trip is normal.

Birth Holistically

This model has also been called the social model. It is about empowering women to have their babies naturally, without interventions and medicine. These people believe that birth is as natural as any other physiological process and that a woman's body is designed to have the baby. Many of these people avoid contacting a doctor and prefer midwives, Doulas and friends for support. To them birth is not an emergency; it is an emergence, a rite of passage, and a family experience.

The model focuses on social factors such as nutrition, rest, exercise, and reducing stress. Surveys across the nation report that doctors spend on average five to ten minutes a prenatal visit, where professionals working with in this holistic model spend at least an hour per appointment. Instead of relying on machines for testing a woman, they use hands-on techniques. The medical model concentrates on the data sheets in front of them: blood tests, urine analysis, sonograms and medical histories. They are the birth engineers, and they are about their readouts, dials, instruments and graphs. The holistic model of care while evaluating the progression of pregnancy focuses on building a support team for the woman and her family for the pregnancy birth and postpartum adjustment.

If your partner believes the following, she will most likely approach birth with a holistic philosophy:

- A mother and her unborn baby are inseparable and interdependent.

- Birth is a mystery.

- Pregnancy is a natural process not to be supplanted by science.

- The emotional, physical, mental and spiritual experiences of life are inseparable.

- Pregnancy and childbirth are intimate, sexual, internal, private events to be shared in an environment with professionals you chose.

- A woman has intuitive knowledge of herself and her baby.

- A woman has the innate ability to nurture her pregnancy and birth her baby and that there is an awesome power and beauty in giving birth.

- Birth is something we can learn from but never control.

- Each woman has responsibility for making choices that are right for her.

- Birth affirms the unity and integrity of family.

- Motherhood is the defining central feature of womanhood.

(*Summarized from Rooks, 1999*)

What is Your Belief System?

You may not really have a strong inclination to either birth philosophy, but you should begin to evaluate your own thinking. It is important to establish a joint philosophy with your partner early on. If you are an adherent of technology, you will generally favor technology and science in birth. If you prefer natural things, choosing a life style that works toward social responsibility, you may favor the holistic belief system. But just as in any theory, religious, political or social, most people fall in between these two "ideals."

The clash between these models is likely to bring about great consternation if a woman endeavors to accomplish birth through an alternative birth philosophy in the hospital other than the medical model. It is no small under taking to consider achieving a natural childbirth in the Birth Machines territory. It involves assuring that the members of your birth team are in agreement with your wishes surrounding your birth in a location outfitted to accommodate the medical model of care. This is why choosing the environment is so extremely important. Let's looks at some of the philosophical differences to better understand why conflicts result.

Birth Machine Rules
- Birth is inherently dangerous
- Pain and trauma can be overcome with drugs

- Birth is the doctor's business
- The husband coaches her with behavioral controlling techniques
- The baby is the doctor's reward for his work
- Birth is a mechanical process
- Birth is controlled by the doctor
- Birth should occur on a set time table
- The doctor delivers the baby

Natural Childbirth
- Birth is inherently trustworthy
- Pain and trauma can be overcome with supportive people
- Birth is a woman's business
- Her attendant gives her emotional support

- The baby is the mother's reward for her work
- Birth is a natural process
- Birth is a process that controls itself
- Birth ebbs and flows

- The mother births the baby

Birth Philosophy Statistics

According to Robbie David Floyd's book "Birth as an American Rite of Passage," women fall about 18% in the medical philosophical model and 6% in the holistic. That leaves 76% who fall in between. The breakdown listed in her book was as follows:

Full acceptance of the medical model

Doctor will take care of everything	9%
Rejecting biology in favor or technology	9%

Full acceptance of the holistic approach

Birth is a natural aspect of womanhood	3%
Birth is a spiritual process of growth	3%

Women in between the two approaches

Maintaining conceptual distance/ natural childbirth in the hospital	15%
Maintaining conceptual distance/ placing technology at the service of the individual	10%
Conceptual fusion with medicine	42%
Conceptual fusion with medicine due to distress	9%

You may not understand that you and your partner have a theoretical basis for the philosophy you approach birth with. Since over 95% of women birth in hospitals, it requires a little bit of extreme thinking on the holistic side to be able to fight the tide and swim upstream to have a birth in a free-standing birth center or at home. Often, the people who chose this route have other beliefs that tend to be more radical and revolutionary as well. Many of these women feel completely let down due to way birth is handled. The more negative their first birth experiences, the more they will buck the system in later births.

Also what is clear is that women, who are in positions of influence and power in government and corporations, chose to have their birth under the medical model so that they can be in control. This means that the ground between these two groups of women can be radically different. Yet the more educated and wealthy women are the more likely that they will choose a midwife or birth center.

Basically the underlying assumption in North American society is that technology is inherently good, and the purveyors of that technology have your best interest at heart. But as discussed, there are many conflicts of interest in that ideology. First there is money in all medicine. Doctors are part of one of the most highly paid professions in society. Ob/gyns are at the top of the doctor salary scale, too. They derive their wealth and livelihood from the work they do. This is not a philanthropic art. As mentioned, more surgeries are performed on women who have good insurance. Why? Because the doctors are assured of being paid handsomely. Women on Medicare rarely get the expensive technological interventions unless they are likely to die if they don't receive emergency help. Studies show that poor minority women are three times more likely to have their babies die, though that may have more to do with social issues like poverty as it relates to nutrition.

Faith is Philosophy: Philosophy is Faith

We have been told that the human body is just a biochemical machine. Our dominant belief system is that science is god-like, so doctors hold the social duty to be priests of these scientific tenets.   American biomedicine's cures are based on science, affected by technology, and carried out in institutions founded on principles of patriarchy and the supremacy of the institution over the individual; however, this viewpoint separates all the moral, spiritual and ethical issues away from the health of an individual.

Most North Americans buy into this philosophy; they have been raised to believe that doctors are next to God in wisdom and authority. In some ways modern medicine has supplanted faith in God. People have learned that medicine can cure anything regardless of the facts. Instead of choosing to believe that God heals, they have been taught to see the doctor and his equipment as their salvation. It seems only the radicals in our society would ever believe that something supernatural or "super natural" could heal. Everyone just expects that our medical priesthood hold the secrets of the arts of healing. This idea doesn't translate well when it comes to birth.

Birth is not something you cut out, burn out, or drug out. Babies are not germs to be eradicated, and the uterus is not a bacterially infested tissue. Babies are not abscesses or abnormal growths or cancers. Whenever the "cut out, burn out, or eradicate" thinking of medicine gets involved, they proceed with the same determination and focus. It is no wonder that their intent is to relieve a woman of this "unnatural" condition. Then compounding the illogical bent is the idea that women are inferior men with imperfect thinking. So the baby and the woman's body are seen as aberrant and something to be repaired.

> The demise of the midwife and the rise of the male-attended, mechanically manipulated birth followed close on the heels of the wide cultural acceptance of the metaphor of the female body as a defective machine -- a metaphor that eventually formed the philosophical foundation of modern obstetrics. Obstetrics was thereby enjoined from its beginnings to develop tools and technologies for the manipulation and improvement of the inherently defective and therefore anomalous and dangerous process of birth. (Davis-Floyd 51)

This poor thinking comes from western history's belief that women are deformed humans and that men are the true models of perfection. This kind of thinking should not surprise us when we realize that this is similar to the thinking that certain Arian races are superior to others. The definition that women are but mutilated males permeates Aristotle's writings, which had a huge impact in the scientific and industrial revolutions. This patriarchal falsehood is part of the male-dominated philosophical background of medicine. Medical literature dealing with women's health issues still to this day highlight a negative view of normal women's bodies. Word like "degenerative," "decay," etc. are often used to describe the normal bodily reproductive processes of a woman's body.

Making Choices

Another issue of philosophical importance is how you make choices during the birth process. You must realize that the birth machine operates still as if you don't have choices. They do not want people meddling with their practices and protocols. But, as you may realize freedom to choose is something that people will die for. You may have to fight to have your say. Learning to advocate for the choices you and your partner want to make is extremely important. Besides, you are the consumer; therefore, you have the right to dictate how your healthcare dollars are going to be spent.

The first choice to be concerned with is whom you can take to the birth. Literature shows that having a labor support person involved reduces interventions like cesareans and epidurals. So if your prospective professional resists at even letting you at the birth, tell them you want to bring another outside party like a Doula and see their reaction. The more they resist the more you know how they will feel if you chose to resist interventions. At times one may encounter a philosophy that discounts the right of patients to exercise their choice in care believing that the patient is ignorant and that they really don't know anything, anyway so why should they have a voice in their care. After all this mindset reasons they have been sought out as an expert for the delivery of care, instead of understanding that health care is a joint venture between the patient and care provider.

Needless to say, the more informed a woman and her partner are, the better opportunity they will have of influencing what choices can be had. If you feel that you lack enough information or experience or fortitude, you definitely will not be able to parley with a doctor. That is why so many people are bringing with them a Doula. Studies show that when a woman goes into the hospital, that her risk of having interventions is lowered when there is a person assisting her continuously through the process of birth. That means greater freedom of keeping control of the birth. Doulas provide emotional support for the birthing mother and assist parents by advocating for the parents desires and wishes for their birth. We must find a way to put the midwife in the hospital and bringing along a Doula for your birth is a huge place to start.

Problems with Philosophies

A study done in 1989 showed that in freestanding birth centers the cesarean rates were 4.4 percent, while the rate was approximately 25% in the hospitals. Researchers have concluded that the difference has to do with philosophies (as in the medical model versus the holistic). It appears that these rates have more to do with where a woman decides to have her baby and what philosophy is dominant in each institution.

Another problem with the medical model is that things are done to benefit the staff at the hospital rather than to ensure the best care. Studies have shown that if the newborn is breastfeed 20 minutes after the birth that there is a lowering of the incidence of infections. Many hospitals still keep the babies from the mother though scientific data shows that there are less Staph (staphylococcal) infections in newborns that spend more than 50% of their time with their mother. The colonization rates of bacteria were twice as high in babies that stayed more than 50% of the time away from their mothers. The second a baby is born the baby has no microorganisms on it. The sterile baby is, however, covered with disease causing germs within five minutes.

Scientific research shows that the early hours after birth are the most important bonding time period. This is another choice hospitals may try to deny you, though science shows the benefit. The mother's breastfeeding begins with a substance that is called colostrums. This thick liquid contains all sorts of vitamins and antibodies from the mother. It is like an elixir of health. Many babies will breastfeed almost instantly after being born – of course, the mucus has to be removed from their mouths and noses first. In the birth machine, it is standard protocol to whisk the baby away, after the birth not pausing to allow skin to skin contact and initiate breastfeeding.

If you allow the hospital professionals to take your baby away, there are other consequences. Separating the baby from your partner can also lead to post partum depression. Make sure you fight for your baby, don't let the doctors or nurses take the baby for any extended length of time unless it is for very clear medical reasons. Whatever needs to be done medically can be done bedside, but the hospital staff for their convenience take the baby to another room for observation if you don't stop them.

Another interesting choice you may want to be aware of is how the whole family is involved. Many families want to celebrate the birth, and as mentioned before that in Greece where pregnant women are put on a pedestal, women who have familial support have better outcomes. However, hospitals may make all sorts of demands that conflict with bringing in family members. In the hospital, you are in is the birth machine's territory. As in the past they even kept fathers out of the birth rooms, they may dissuade any other family members from entering the labor and delivery rooms. Yet, if you and your partner desire to share birth with your family, let it be known up front.

Collaborative Care: When Flight Plans Change

There are times that a woman with a strong bent toward holistic care for whatever reason finds herself in a position where the desires of her heart a natural childbirth are contraindicated and flight plans will need to change. Does this mean that she may not receive holistic health care, or receive the nurture and guidance of a midwife for her prenatal and birth care? Absolutely not!

It is the mark of the model for maternity care that obstetricians and midwives work together in what is known as collaborative care. Dr. G. J. Kloosterman was a frame worker of the Netherlands Maternity Health Codes and Chief of Obstetrics and Gynecology at the University of Amsterdam. Dr. Kloosterman is passionate about the need for both the midwife and obstetrician to be able to practice alongside one another to deliver the highest level of maternity care. His ardent belief is that we need both practitioners and that the midwife needs the obstetrician just as much as the obstetrician needs the midwife. Dr. Kloosterman writes "Throughout the world, there exists a group of women who feel mightily drawn to giving care to women in childbirth. At the same time maternal and independent, responsive to a mother's needs, yet accepting full responsibility as her attendant; such women are natural midwives.

Without the presence and acceptance of the midwife, obstetrics becomes aggressive, technical, and inhuman."

It is the law in Britain that midwives are the primary provider of maternity care and that they are legally bound to attend all births wherever they occur. If a complication occurs prenatally or at a birth and the care needs to be transferred to an obstetrician, the midwife is duty bound to continue her care and attend her birth. So legally in Britain an obstetrician cannot deliver a baby without the presence of a midwife. Such an arrangement is not limited to the UK. Midwives and physicians can work well together in the United States as well, and the more professional they are the greater likelihood that they will work well together.

If you and your partner face a scenario where the birth sincerely necessitates the skills of an obstetrician, where you have been risked out of traditional midwifery care, your midwife should be able to refer you to an accommodating obstetrician, most likely someone that she has worked with previously. At the same time there are many progressive physicians who count among their colleagues some midwives that they have developed a professional rapport with and you and your partner could discuss with your physician the inclusion of midwifery care in your prenatal and birth care.

When one experiences disappointment, it is difficult not to lose focus. It is important to remember that though your expectations for the birth have been upset you need not lose everything. A helpful thing to do is to take inventory and determine what aspect of the birth expectation seemed most important to you and your partner. For some couples it is discovering the sex of their baby for themselves without having a jubilant birth attendant announce it to them. For others it is that they be allowed to give their baby its first bath after the birth. Whatever the aspect of the expected birth is relevant to you may still be preserved even though you have to contend with a higher level of care. Birth attendants can be prepared to hand you the baby for you to observe for yourselves whether you have a boy or girl, and arrangements can be made to have a warm tub of water available in the delivery room for you to enjoy bathing your baby yourselves. The important thing is to identify what is the piece of the birth that you had imagined was to be the most meaningful and begin with your health care providers to explore how you may still retain that special piece of the birth for your family. It can be done!

Birth Techniques Based on These Philosophies

Several types of birthing techniques are popular in North America. Lamaze is by far the preferred method – it is highly supported by hospitals and most of medicine. The Bradley method is still taught around the country, and is drawn on holistic theories. There are a variety of other methods, some which focus on hypnosis, some that relate to alternative medicine like acupuncture, massage, etc. All methods draw from a philosophical root.

Lamaze which trains a woman to use breathing to control her behavior during childbirth became the favorite method since it falls within the ritual acceptable practice of the birth machine. The Lamaze breathing focus helps a woman to enhance her mind body separation. Lamaze instructors are even hired by hospitals. Lamaze is so popular that it often shows up in our movies and television episodes.

The Bradley method doesn't teach your partner to be a compliant patient, unquestioning and uninformed. Bradley believes that there are natural principles involved in childbirth. Dr. Bradley was in attendance at over 14,000 births, of which 94% were intervention free and unmedicated. The philosophy is holistic essentially. Bradley stresses mind body integration. Bradley instructors are often harassed or barely tolerated by hospital staff since they discourage women from taking drugs and other interventions.

Many birthing techniques are designed to foster a more cooperative patient for the birth machine. This is especially true of Lamaze. When your partner has practiced hour after hour of their breathing exercises, this promotes the type of behavior that functions best for the hospital staff. The idea is to have you coach her through so that she never loses emotional control. As long as she is controlling her behavior then she is out of the way of whatever the hospital staff wants.

So consider carefully what philosophy and technique line up with you and your partner's philosophy, then you will be fine.

Stress Brings Out the True Philosophy

Depending on your overall beliefs, you will head into the type of birth you want thinking that you have it mastered. However, any plan you have may hit rough and turbulent skies especially if you birth in a stressful environment. Then the real philosophy your partner has will come out.

Many women really don't have a clear philosophical viewpoint heading into birth. They have ideas of what they would like; but until there is pressure you may not see the real personality of your partner come out immediately. Those who are likely to argue with a sales clerk about damaged merchandize may already be a self-advocating type. However, if your partner tends to follow in conversations and activities, and not express herself with much force, she may follow the dictates of others, especially authoritative types. The quote "As a woman Lives, so shall she birth, so shall she die." widely circulated in the seventy's and published in Gayle Peterson's and Lewis Mehl-Madrona's book titled <u>Birthing Normally: A Personal Growth Approach to Childbirth</u> says it all. Birth brings out something in all women. Women tell us that each birth brings out something different, and that they often learn more about themselves in the process.

The point here is that when stress occurs, it can suddenly draw out or undermine your partner's philosophy. Stress affects cognition. When a person is not stressed they have the ability to view the world from a broad and abstract perspective -- allowing one to judge situations on their own merits. But with tremendous stress, an individual may only be able to choose between either-or options, seeing the world as only black or white. If the stress doesn't relent, then the person can fall into disorientation and mental disintegration. The physiological process of labor is itself stressful. The added noise, bustle, and continual interference in a hospital environment multiple that stress. The more stressful it gets the more your partner is not going to be able to make good decisions and the more she is going to feel like she has totally lost control, driving her to give up her philosophical position and her autonomy and to only say yes to whoever is working with her.

Everyone reacts differently to stress. Some people are driven by it and others are afraid to act. That is why some women choose to align their philosophical views with the birth machine once they get into the hospital; this is not a conscious decision, but one forced upon them. Genny recalls when giving birth to our second child after explicit direction to the labor unit that there were to be no observers to the birth, a chipper student entered the birth room and announced that she would be watching the birth of our child, adding would that be ok? Genny continues, "I was just about to begin pushing our daughter out and all my energy was focused on that. I could not invest my strength in a dialog with this person standing at the door in my position of being in the intense throws of birth work. A simple 'yes' was all I could articulate. Fortunately for me Phil and I had a labor support person with us, and she intervened and said to the woman I don't believe that she, referring to me wants to have any student observers, 'isn't that right, Genny' she asked?" All I had to do was nod my head and return quickly to the work that lay ahead. Our labor support provider had saved the day!

Women may also actually find it easier to just submit to the routines and hospital protocols once there. If a woman is too stressed to articulate what she wants, someone else has to, and, if you don't, the birth machine will do what they want regardless of your beliefs. Your partner needs to not have to deal with distractions or fights; she has enough to do. It is your job to hire someone to fight for her needs or for you to be assertive yourself. It has been said putting women in the position of coping with conflict when they should be concentrating on having their babies is counted as an intervention itself. For some women falling into the hands of the coercive birth machine is positive. They like it because they don't have to think. The machine makes all the decisions for them. This reliance on ritual gives many people a sense of safety. It's like other rituals they've grown up with – they are taught to believe the rituals by the larger culture.

Birth Philosophy Conflict

Depending on your partner's expectations, birth can be a wonderful and joyful experience. If you have ever heard women talk about this, you will find that the birth philosophy a woman has sets her course for the experience. If she buys into the superiority of man's technology, then she will want every part of the hospital birth. Her experience will be channeled by these expectations and the affect the birth machine has in controlling her. The best type of birth preparation for such a birth would be childbirth education classes in the hospital – most likely free. Agreeing with the birth machine will only reduce your partner's stress levels when birthing there. When a woman has both the holistic and the technocratic philosophies in mind, you will see that she is confused about what she wants. That is why writing out that birth plan is useful. Removing contradictions in our thinking helps us to focus and proceed.

If your partner is holistic in her approach, then you will find that trying to go for it in the hospital will be nothing but conflict – unless you are able to find a holistic midwife or doctor to protect your partner's desires. That is why the statistics show that women have better outcomes when they have a labor support person working with them through the whole birth process. These people are constantly intervening with the hospital staff, trying to reduce unnecessary interventions and procedures if that is what you want.

Ultimately learning what birth philosophy you and your partner have is crucial. Identifying the environment that aligns to that idea is essential in setting the stage for the birth you have chosen.

Remember your mission – you are there to help her have the best birth possible. If you and your partner have different viewpoints, all you can do to keep your relationship at peace is to inform. Many men try to interfere with a woman's autonomy. But as the character of God said in Bruce Almighty, love must come from free will. Though you may have the best of intentions for your partner, and that is obvious because you have even taken the time to read this book, you must let her make the choices. Support her choices and tenderly influence her, but most of all affirm her.

Birth Facility Philosophy

We dare say that most people make the decision of where they birth and who they birth with based primarily on money. "Where will the insurance allow the birth and which doctors do I have to choose from?" Some insurance companies will pay for freestanding birth centers and even home birth. Genny and Phil were able in the 1990s to convince Blue Cross of Indiana to let them use a freestanding birth center. Kaiser in California uses a lot of midwives at their facilities. Make sure the facilities you head toward are supportive of your birth philosophy.

Remember the doctors and the hospitals may have different birth philosophies as well. Staff at those medical institutions may also not share the same philosophies. However, the natural childbirth movement did impact hospitals. Freestanding birth center also arose from that movement. The hospitals themselves did not change their philosophies much after this; they did, however add specially decorated rooms called birthing suites to address the demands of their birth consumers.

Birthing Suites

Trying to create the perfect balance between safety and ardently stated desires of many women for "control" and "natural childbirth," hospitals across the nation began during the late 1970s and early 1980s to provide "alternative birth centers" and "birthing suites." These birthing centers were the medical profession's answer to the consumer demands of women scarred by their experiences in regular labor and delivery, and to the many sympathetic nurses and doctors who sincerely sought to provide something better. With their attractive décor, privacy, kitchenette, big double bed, and open doors to family and friends, they seemed to represent the perfect mediation of the holistic/technocratic dichotomy for many couple (Birthrite 185).

Fitting in with the Medical Model

What the Birth Machine wants from men is *compliance*. They want you to be part of the process as long as they can use you to ensure their type of birth is guaranteed. Coleman Romalis writing in his book "Taking Care of the Little Women" states that the father at birth often allows the hospital to co-opt him in favor of the birth machine and then to utilize his influence to further the alignment of his wife's perceptions to that philosophy. Many women, who have already had previous births, have told me that they don't want their partners involved in birth because they interfere with their autonomy. The hospitals know that they can use the male partner to bend the will of the mother to their ways. Just be aware that they may try to use you to contradict the philosophy of your partner. If you have not taken the time to determine your own philosophical stance, then you may be easily influenced. You need to stand with your own convictions throughout the labor and delivery. Remember you need to focus on supporting and strengthening your partner's philosophy in this whole affair. Don't be manipulated!

The messages underlying the birth machine's workings are that the institution is all powerful, that pregnant women are sick and frail, that women can't birth naturally because their bodies are defective and that to save everyone the hassle surgery is a painless way of having the baby.

The medical or Cartesian model of the body-as-machine operates to make the physician a technician, or mechanic. The body breaks down and needs repair, it can be repaired in the hospital as a car is in the shop; once fixed the person can be returned to the community. The earliest models in medicine were largely mechanical; later models worked more with chemistry, and newer, more sophisticated medical writing describes the body as programmed and computer-like, but the basic point remains the same. Problems in the body are technical problems requiring technical solutions (Rothman 1982:34).

Philosophy Counterattacks

When you and your partner agree as to what philosophy you are going to be holding when "you are pregnant," you will find the world has its own perspective and views, and the strong willed will try to impose their ideas on you too, especially if they "wish the best for you." Irritating family members will tell you everything about their experience with birth and make sure you agree with them. Birth is your experience, so you may need to learn some buffering techniques. You must make sure that you don't take a negative position against people who truly love your partner, but at the same time you can't support their philosophies if they contradict hers. This is the type of conflict management for senior peace negotiators.

The "doctor is always right" camp and the holistic folks will have opinions that they may try and force-feed you. This again shows how you have to be prepared to advocate for your partner's chosen belief system, screening out the negative. This conflict is something to be prepared for. We suggest screening out those who continuously assault you partner's ideology. Do not let others browbeat you partner. If you don't, your partner may be torn between pleasing herself and pleasing her "benefactors." Such indecisiveness is historically the cause of disasters.

After a birth, when you both are spent, these benefactors tend to take advantage of the situation, and begin to impose their will, trying to help you out. You must keep alert and insure that things are copasetic for you partner. Remember she may be extremely weakened by her birth especially if she had any surgery, blood loss or infection. Protect her and your baby's right to breastfeed, as breastfeeding has its own benefits for the mother and baby.

Ground Operations: Breast Feeding

You may wonder why breast feeding is important: First it benefits the mother. You need to understand that a uterus has to return to its normal size after the childbirth; this is called involution. Remember that organ the uterus started out on the other side of the pregnancy about the size of an orange and has blossomed to the size of a watermelon. When a mother breastfeeds, the uterus begins clamping down, causing further involution, reduced blood loss, and cramps for the mother (called after pains). The cramping is more significant for later pregnancies.

Your place may be to be emotionally supportive during these changes and cramping. Be tender and understanding, if you can. Remind her that she is accomplishing a magnificent thing by feeding her baby and having her uterus return to its pre pregnancy state.

The second benefits are the many advantages that breastfeeding offers the baby.

When we study breast milk we are amazed at what is known as specifity. Breast milk is constantly changing to meet the needs of the baby, and it is specific for the time of delivery. The breast milk a mother produces is different for a premature baby and a full term baby. It is like the body knows just how to manufacture the type of milk the baby needs and as the baby grows the breast milk changes to meet the demands of that stage of development. Breast milk for a newborn, a three month old and a six month old are all composed differently. The woman's body knows intrinsically how to produce breast milk to meet the needs of her individual child. Breast milk is the best thing to feed to a premature baby.

Breastfeeding has countless benefits to the baby and to the family however, we recognize that not everyone will be able to breastfeed or even desire to breastfeed, if this is where you and your partner are. You must diligently affirm that your partner is being the best mother to your child and that feeding methods have little to do with demonstrating the capacity of love and care one has for their child. It is in the feeding and caring for the child that her love is demonstrated and you may have to negate messages from breastfeeding enthusiasts that might suggest otherwise.

If you and your mate believe that you want your child to breast feed, then the place to begin is during the pregnancy. The best advice we ever received on breast feeding came from Bill and Martha Sears and we echo that same advice to you. Attend a series of meeting of La Leche League International while you are expecting before the birth. La Leche League is an organization that provides education, information and peer support for breastfeeding. The organization covers four topics on breastfeeding on an ongoing basis. Because of the discretion with breastfeeding it predominantly is a woman only organization, however from time to time they will host a couple's session or have a special couple's night where you can go and participate with other fathers.

Having your partner attending these meetings can help her learn about breastfeeding and prevent problems from occurring or to learn how to handle problems when they come up. Attendance should begin well in advance before the birth to create the best knowledge base for your partner before the baby comes. Our experience with attending La Leche League meetings with our first pregnancy proved to established breastfeeding for us. Oftentimes a woman will not only find the breastfeeding education necessary to nurse through La Leche League but will also find a support system for herself and her young family while fostering friends and relationships for years to come. Guys usually have no clue on how important this component in life is.

A wealth of studies proves hands down that breastfeeding and breast milk are the best method of feeding a baby and the best thing to feed a baby. However mothers who choose to breastfeed are still being criticized for their choice from those with a different philosophical perspective. Whole generations of women were taught that formula is better and a more superior method of feeding than breast feeding. They are simply ignorant of how much better breast milk and breast feeding is for a child. As bad as ignorance is, things can get ugly when one tries to force their views on another. It is unfortunate that there are some people who erroneously believe that parents who breastfeed their children do not have the best interest of the child at heart. They believe somehow that the desire of a woman to breastfeed her child is selfish, and that she should be ensuring that the child receive the nutrients that formula offers. What they do not understand is that breast milk is the best and most complete nutrition for the child! Men need to be encouraging to their mates and supportive of their choices. You need to be the strong one here and realize the large influence that you carry with your mate, and make sure she know what an awesome job she is doing. We are aware of countless stories where the father's words of encouragement and support made the difference between a successful breastfeeding relationship and one that ended with disappointment. Be ready to counterattack a society that is not supportive of breastfeeding and advocate for your mate and your child's right to establish breastfeeding in the birth machine, and for the right to carry on an ongoing breastfeeding relationship.

Interventions Can Stop Her Progress

For the women who want to have their babies with as little intervention as possible, or in other words those expecting a natural childbirth, certain interventions can completely eliminate those choices. This holds particularly true for epidural anesthesia; its safety protocols prohibit most of the practices used in natural childbirth. Once you make a choice to deviate from your birth plan, you will be forced to do what comes next. Medical interventions lead to more interventions.

Conclusion

Birth philosophies are extremely important in formulating a good birth plan. Having a birth philosophy that lines up with who you birth with will make the childbirth much easier to handle. If your partner and you have different philosophies, this can cause relational problems. Choices you make for where you birth, who you birth with and who you allow at the birth all should be based on you and your partner's philosophical beliefs. Remember birth is one of the pinnacle moments in a woman's life, so eliminating certain conflicts ahead of time will improve the overall satisfaction!

Chapter 13: Entering the Birth Machine

Since 99 percent of North American women birth in medical hospitals, the birth machine is the experience of most women, so you will most likely be headed for a hospital-based birth. As this book has pointed out, if your partner believes in the medical perspective, then you are safest in that environment psychologically, but as you have learned in this book, the notion that birth is safer in a hospital is a just a myth. Medical literature itself shows that the standards of care used today are intrinsically risky. Active management of labor forces labor to speed up and become more dangerous, painful and stressful.

U.S. Department of Health Statistics shows that the rates for interventions continue to rise. In 2002 they reported the highest recorded rates of cesarean sections ever. Inductions, use of the Electronic Fetal Monitor, Inductions and Episiotomies are now routine procedures. Most of these interventions are unnecessary medically in low risk pregnancies and increase the cost of birth dramatically. However, despite all these facts, you may end up choosing to follow the majority and have your baby in the hospital.

Medical Perspective

The birth machine is programmed by obstetrics. Obstetricians are specialty medical doctors who study the pathology of women's reproductive organs, and who are trained as surgeons. They are supposed to work to save your partner and baby. They say that they will aggressively prevent any danger from happening, using all of their knowledge and technology to stop bad things from happening.

Unfortunately, it is these attitudes about birth that have promoted over use of tests and interventions. They use the techniques developed for high-risk pregnancies on low risk pregnancies. You would think that birth is like having a coronary.

Medicine should be based on scientific experience and wisdom. Control studies should determine the safety and effectiveness of clinical procedures. Obviously institutionalized medical practices, "the ways of the birth machine," defy logic and scientific fact. The aggressive management of childbirth that is designed to provide a high level of safety doesn't follow what the scientific studies show and prove. Outdated routines are supported rather than developing new safer approaches. This is especially true for the use of certain interventions as mentioned before.

Medicine is a huge business, and birth is a big part of that pie. Therefore those who control the industry have a lot to lose if they change their practices, making them less invasive and less technological. If you have a brand new $20,000 dollar piece of equipment at your hospital, and it measures the progress of birth, you use it. Who cares if auscultation is more accurate?

The medical perspective is favor institutional factors over individual desire in its perspective. The birthing mother becomes an object and a patient, not actively controlling the experience. And that is what you need to know if you have your children in that environment.

Let's become acquainted with the birth machine's general practices under the "active management" concepts. If you know what to expect, then you can better be prepared for the real thing. Think of it as watching game films before the big game.

Getting to the Hospital

Following the normal procedures of many hospitals, when you and your partner arrive at the hospital, she is placed in a wheelchair. They wheel her to the labor and delivery room. The nurses begin the prep work after the basic paperwork is completed. Your partner is undressed of her own clothing and placed in hospital garb that doesn't cover her body effectively – a psychological way of reducing her to the bottom rung in the power structure (think of it as being a soldier in basic training – the regime reduces you to the lowest of low). Then an enema is offered and possibly the shaving her pubic hair (for possible surgery). A heparin lock or an IV is applied next. She is then placed back in a bed to go through early labor. In some cases, the doctor may be in the building and will come check in on you. If the doctor isn't available and the labor is in its early stages, you may not see the doctor for hours – especially if it is during the week and the doctor's office is miles away. The nurses keep them informed.

If labor is progressing quickly or too quickly (precipitously), you may see another, unknown doctor at the door. This usually means that your doctor is not going to work with you on this delivery. Regardless, the nursing staff or possible a nurse-midwife, if such a practitioner is working there, will check to see where your partner's labor is standing – this is determined by a vaginal exam -- to see how much she has dilated and effaced. The cervix is measured to see how wide and open it is.

Very Early Labor

When your partner is in the beginning of her labor, she will be less than 5 centimeters dilated. This stage of labor is slow going and sometimes lasts more than 24 to 36 hours – especially from 1 to 4 centimeters dilation. The hospital staff usually will not do anything but check on you very periodically to determine whether the labor is effectively opening the cervix. You may feel abandoned, but remember they usually have many other mothers birthing down the hall. Early labor in the hospital is a time of waiting and hoping that things will move forward smoothly, but in first-time mothers, this usually doesn't happen that way – first labors are on average much longer than any subsequent births.

At some point, either labor dies down or heats up. But generally the first stage is long and slow. Often first-time mothers (nulliparous women) will go to the hospital before the labor really engages since the new feelings of labor are so odd and disconcerting. They usually go because they are stressed or excited and want reassurance.

The birth machine will try to speed up labor by breaking the bag of waters (amniotomy) when nothing is happening – which is very common. The cervix may efface and not open for literally a couple of days.

At first there is no real concern unless the waters have broken.

Broken Bag of Waters

Once the bag of waters breaks, a chance exists for infection. Infections can kill (especially underdeveloped) babies and should be avoided. Amniotomy is a medical means of breaking the waters to hurry the birth process up. The birth machine will usually not give a woman more than 24 hours to have her baby once the waters have broken even if they force it to happen. They usually start induction agents at the halfway point.

Induction and Augmentation

Oxytocin is generally administered for those failing to progress or to those whose waters have broken. This is to help open the cervix, but unless the cervix has been chemically or naturally prepared beforehand this procedure will not affect that change. Doctors will administer a cervix-softening agent, but this too can add to the power of contractions. If the cervix is ready, the stimulating drug oxytocin (pitocin is the synthesized version and is called Pit by hospital staff). Oxytocin is the chemical that triggers the muscles in the uterus to open things up. The birth machine generally gives a woman twice (or more) the ordinary physiologically produced level of oxytocin.

When oxytocin is administered, and when you are in a hospital that has a busy maternity ward, the Electronic Fetal Monitor (EFM) is going to be brought out. This machine is supposed to register when there are troubles with the baby or mother. This usually requires a woman to remain on her back through labor, which invariable slows birth down by eliminating oxygen flow to the uterus and the placenta (thereby reducing the oxygen to the baby which can trigger fetal distress). New equipment has been designed for vertical movement, but still the machine is a ball-and-chain weight on motion.

Once oxytocin and other inducers are hooked up (some inducers are directly applied to the cervix to rapidly ripen it), your partner may find that her contractions get very painful and powerful. This puts most women in a scary position. To me it's like cooking eggs in a frying pan. If you cook the eggs slowly, they don't burn. Turn up the heat, and you have to be highly diligent not to burn them. The hospital does not want birth to slow down and that burner to be turned off. It wastes their time for one thing. Then for every hour you are in the birth suite and under the care of staff costs the hospital money.

As we've said, oxytocin is supposed to get the labor on track – studies show it saves about an hour on average in the first stage of labor. But once those waters are broken, there are several things that all can happen that push the birth into more risky situations.

Cascading Interventions

First, since an unripe cervix is not going to open and the contractions get really hard to bear labor becomes hard and painful, but effects no positive physical change in the birth canal. Here are a few of the things that can happen:

- The birth machine will start dispensing drugs to ease the increased pain

- The woman will become discouraged if her labor isn't progressing

- Hypertension will distress the baby

- An infection can occur to both baby and mother, since the waters have been broken

- The mother can become exhausted, since long painful labors wear a woman out

- The mother will be hooked to the EFM, which has a high level of inaccurate readings, some that miss real dangers, others that show real danger but too late, and more often than not show danger when there isn't any problem.

- The baby will have a probe stuck into its head – this is to get a more clear reading of fetal heart rates but further adds to the chance of maternal and infant infection

Epidurals

Next usually comes the epidural. This procedure requires an injection of drugs into the spine to deaden the pain of labor. Many women, once they are riding the forceful contractions of oxytocin, will feel like the contractions are unbearable to the point of psychologically rattling them. The epidural for many women saves the day, for others it kills their contractions. Epidurals will either set someone up to kill their progress or help a woman get back in control. So if it kills progress, the birth machine has basically run its non-surgical means of forcing labor – surgery will be next. If a woman gets back in control, isn't exhausted and without juice (remember they usually won't let her eat even after hours of labor), then she may be able to have the baby vaginally, but since she can't feel anything, she can't tell when the baby is coming and when she has to push. This sets up the episiotomy. This is another procedure routinely done to women without need.

Emergency Cesarean Surgery

Now if there are signs that the mother is becoming exhausted or the baby is showing signs of fetal distress, be ready to scrub up and go to OR (the operating room). This is going to happen in over 27% of first-time mothers (Menacker 2005), 39% of breech presentations, and 80% of VBAC (vaginal birth after cesarean) attempts. The better your insurance and the more expensive the hospital you are in, the higher chance you face of having surgery – the cesarean is the most often performed major surgery in the US. Remember, doctors usually speak of a vaginal birth as a trial of labor – they let your partner **try** to have a vaginal birth. They would be just as happy to hand you a baby without all this trouble. They have fought insurance companies for years and won the right to provide elected c-sections. That means your partner just schedules her birth for Monday at 9 am – or whenever the doctor has a free slot on his schedule. Surgery is profitable and easy for surgeons.

Men's Place in the Machine

Most guys spend their time in the hospital not knowing what to do. They don't know why things are done they way they are, and they don't question what is being done. They basically just sit there and watch the EFM strips showing the coming contractions. Many guys say it is basically boring and that they are left most of the time with their partner alone. Many guys at their first birth are nervous and anxious without their doctor being around. As mentioned earlier, this is not a good situation as a tense man can cause a woman to be stressed and that prolongs labor. A woman needs to be at peace and undisturbed as labor progresses. Doctors usually don't spend much time with a birthing mother until she is ready to deliver, so that leaves hours with only a few short appearances of the nursing staff. If this is the choice you made, then learn the role of servant like the Doula.

As long as you don't try to stop the machine, you basically have nothing much to do. As long as you don't make waves or contradict your partner, you are fine. You could do that watching a professional game on TV. You could read a novel – remember you have hours. You could just get out of their way. BUT!!!!! Your partner may expect your continuous emotional support. No one else in the birth machine is going to be there for her 24/7. If you go to the birth, expect to be there for hours and hours. You will be offered breaks by the staff, but beware, when your partner is in labor, and no one is with her but the hospital staff, they may try to cajole her into anything they want. If you leave your partner alone, you have just opened the door for anything the birth machine wants to do.

Stopping the Interventions

If you are in the hospital, there are some things you can do to reduce, perhaps stop the interventions. However, remember that the machine is programmed. It will move the conveyor belt forward. Anything that gets in the way is chewed up and spit out, including the partners of laboring women. Now if your partner likes the birth machine, then you only have to be emotionally supportive. Just don't think the machine is programmed for a natural birth plan; no it is programmed for profits.

As Robbie Davis Floyd wrote in her book "Birth as an American Rite of Passage," most women are not philosophically aligned when they get to the hospital. So if you are caring, help your partner to have the birth you understand her to want. If she says no interventions, then you need to take positive steps to reduce the likelihood of those interventions. Hospital birth is going to be about interventions. Birthing with midwives in the hospital is going to lower that chance. Using a Doula is going to lower the rate as well, but there are difficulties since they have no authority in the birth machines territory. Birthing outside of the birth machine is best by far.

Yet, let's look at what you can do to eliminate interventions while in the birth machine. Before any intervention is offered, you have a legal right to know the medical reason for the use. We recommend taking a notebook with you into the birth to note any interventions suggested, why they were suggested and why you refused or accepted them. Remember you (or another support person like a Doula) need to be handling this, not a laboring woman – she fighting for her will only interfere with her labor.

EFM (electronic fetal monitor)

One of the chief impediments to the progress of labor is continuous EFM. It is not in the design of labor and birth for a healthy woman to be restricted to a bed such is necessary for continuous EFM to occur. We can borrow from Native American wisdom their knowledge, "If you lay down, the baby will never come out." A woman needs to be up and vertical for labor to progress. Being vertical and up and moving is simply incompatible with continuous EFM. We encourage you to negotiate with your caregivers the options of monitoring the baby's well being with intermittent auscultation (simply recording the fetal heart rate by listening to it with the aid of a fetoscope or Doppler). The Doppler from the EFM itself can be held on your partners' abdomen by a staff member or you for a quick check on the fetal heart rate. Another possibility is to agree to an initial strip for five to ten minutes upon arriving in labor and delivery. If the expectation for EFM continues you can try to see if monitoring a few moments throughout the labor on the EFM will accommodate the birth machines need for documentation, allowing the majority of time for the laboring woman to be free to move about and find what ever position is working best for her labor, without being tethered down to the EFM.

Consider these things when contemplating your mate being on an EFM. In a group of high risk pregnancies the use of the EFM was found to have no benefit to the mother or baby but doubled or tripled the cesarean section rate. The professor and chairman of the Department of Obstetrics and Gynecology at Harvard Medical School has expressed that the EFM has been a "failed technology" (Ryan 1998).

Amniotomy

Amniotomy or the artificial rupture of membranes (AROM) is a surgical procedure where the amniotic sac is ruptured by a small instrument with a hook on the end. The amniotic sac is ruptured by passing a hook through the cervix and piercing the bag of waters. This is done in an attempt to speed up labor or to look at the amniotic fluid. Avoid going to the hospital in early labor, but when you and your partner get to the hospital, try and steer around this procedure in order to accelerate labor. Remember the 24-hour rule! . By avoiding amniotomy in early labor where the risks are greater for a cord prolapse, you also avoid the internal electronic fetal monitor and, which requires an electrode to be stuck into your baby's head.

Ask a bunch of questions. Ask what potential side effects of the procedure are. Discuss the pros and cons. There are times when birth is eminent, once the woman is complete *(fully dilated)* and pushing that the rupturing of the membranes is beneficial. Note, however, the timing is when the birth is about to happen. There are instances where a mother is completely dilated and pushing over intact membranes and not making any progress, when the membranes are ruptured the baby almost descends immediately. The reason for this is that pushing over an intact bag of membranes requires greater exertion of pressure from the mother than pushing a baby when the membranes are ruptured. Be proactive in the care of your partner and understand where in the timing of the labor the procedure is being recommended and whether or not the benefits out way the risks. Then make an informed decision with your partner.

Use of oxytocin or pitocin to augment labor

Many practitioners will use pitocin or oxytocin to speed up a slow labor, but labor slows down for a variety of reasons. Oxytocin is delivered through an IV usually. Doctors use this and often cause the contractions to get too strong. Being at the hospital too early is generally the problem. False labor and slow labor are common for women who are having their first child – their bodies aren't accustomed to birthing. Think of it, it's like her having a part of herself she has never tried out before. So the first time she births, she may have a lot to learn. But to avoid medically speeding up the labor, try some of the following techniques:

- Pelvic rocking
- Walking or light dancing
- Getting on a fours or squatting (unless knee problems or varicose veins)
- Eating or Drinking (to reduce fatigue)
- Massage and acupuncture
- Warm showers or baths
- Nipple stimulation to produce oxytocin, the natural form of pitocin

Pain Medication

Modern medicine promotes drugs for everything. This is part and parcel of the way all health issues are addressed. You need, or your partner's Doula needs, to be vigilant. Your partner may zone out and accept anything from the health care providers at the birth. Remember she is going through a momentous experience. She may not be able to consciously make decisions on her own. The longer the labor and the more difficult, the less she can fend off the drugs. Avoiding narcotics and analgesics also protects your baby from suffering the effects of the medicines.

The most common analgesia used during labor is Meperidine Pethidine. It is at its highest levels in the baby for 1 to 5 hours after the mother received the drug. This timing is important when considering receiving this pain relief in the labor. Is the birth expected within 1 to 5 hours, or is the medication being recommended to a woman in an exhausted state who is going to take a break from labor and rest for several hours before giving birth? The affects of analgesia transferred through the placenta on the baby are a lowered heart rate before birth. If the baby has the medication in its system after the birth results include lowered Apgar scores, respiratory depression, and a lowered state of alertness which inhibits sucking and causes a delay in effective feeding. Another pain medication sometimes used is Fentanyl; it provides a rapid pain relief with a shorter active duration than Meperidine.

If the labor is advanced 8 – 9 cms dilated it seems prudent to have your mate attempt these alternative techniques for coping with pain before settling for being medicated.

To avoid this, try some of the following techniques:

- Changing Positions
- Presence of continuous labor support Doula other supportive person
- Human Touch back rubs and massage
- Warm water tub or shower
- Encouraging news about her progress
- Heat / cold
- Saline injections in the lower back to reduce back pain (intradermal water blocks)

Epidural

An epidural is a way to offer pain relief during labor. An injection of anesthetic is delivered in the epidural space (located above the sacrum) of the mother's back. This injection acts by blocking the sensations in the spinal nerves. Receiving an epidural may cause a sudden drop in maternal blood pressure and a higher chance of necessitating delivery by instruments, forceps or vacuum extraction or cesarean section. An epidural has been found to increase the need for a cesarean section by two to three times in a mother giving birth for the first time. Frequently there is a malposition of the baby's head because of the relaxed pelvic muscles of the mother, caused by this medication. The mothers lose the ability to coordinate pushing with contractions because she has lost the sensation of the contractions. Forceps and vacuum extraction are not without their own risks of injury to the baby. Epidurals are also associated with a longer length of second stage of labor and the development of a fever in the mother. Epidural anesthesia increases the use of pitocin to augment labor. Furthermore, the baby may experience alternations in the fetal heart rate with the epidural and if the mother develops a fever it means the likelihood of a newborn septic work up including IV antibiotics and isolation in the nursery.

To avoid an epidural utilize all the alternative techniques for relieving pain previously mentioned and get your partner walking. Keep her from getting exhausted. Stay at home as long as possible – like until she reaches five centimeters. If you arrive at the hospital before 5 cms you can always leave and return when labor is more active. Keep your partner energized with nutritious snacks and drinks. Remember labors can last for a couple days. This is an endurance event.

Episiotomy

A complete discussion regarding episitomy is found in chapter 11. To avoid this surgery, you should refuse it as a routine procedure. Make this known at the beginning of your stay in the labor and delivery room. Well before you get to the birth and labor, have your partner do the following:

- Pelvic Floor Contractions (also known as Kegels)
- Prenatal perineal massage
- Avoid Epidurals
- Help her to remember to push when she gets the natural urge only, and to push like the baby is being breathed out (this allows the tissues to fan out)
- Avoid arbitrary time limits set for vacuum extraction of forceps delivery

Cesarean Section

To avoid this surgical procedure, you should stay away from the following

- Early Artificial Rupture of Membranes
- Epidurals
- Induction (Pitocin)
- Cytotec
- Early arrival at the hospital
- Narcotics

Basically, three out of ten births in the hospital end at OR. If you really want to avoid this surgery, then have your babies outside of the hospital, at home or a birth center or if at a hospital with a Doula and carefully selected caregivers.

Chapter 14: Money and Birth

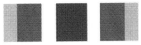

Marsden Wagner, an obstetrician himself and well-known author and expert on birth, wrote a book called "Pursuing the Birth Machine" which details the current birth industry and its focus on interventions. He explains why doctors chose to use risky procedures rather than to let birth occur naturally. The combination of doctors' being afraid to be sued and medicine's desire to make birth financially lucrative has created an environment in which birth is very unnatural and medically controlled. Most people do not realize the huge impact economics has in affecting how birth is handled in North America.

Bread and Butter of Medicine

Since maternity wards are the financial rich centers and the bread and butter of hospitals, the medical community has a lot at stake in selling birth. Tonya Jamois, president of ICAN, International Cesarean Awareness Network reports "Obstetricians and hospitals have found that high-intervention birth warranted or not, is very profitable. So there is a tremendous financial incentive to bypass the clinically optimal approach, and opt for convenience and profits. For example, many hospitals across the country have eliminated facility-based midwifery practices simply because the low –intervention approach, while clinically sound, does not bring in as many dollars."

The average percentage of yearly revenues of a hospital that are generated in the maternity ward is 20%. Hospitals have gone under without having a prospering maternity ward. Birth is a very profitable business, and obstetrical doctors average $275,000 per year. Their professional publications advertise Leer Jets and other luxuries. It was estimated several years ago that this industry brought in yearly over 40 billion dollars for the medical community – that figure is said to have doubled in the past ten years. There were around 35,000 obstetricians, so they commanded about $9.6 billion annually. Hospitals, which took about 55% of the revenue from births, took in around $22.1 billion annually. These figures are based on U.S. Department of Health Services statistics for birth in 1999 from an article that appeared in the Journal of Nurse-Midwifery written by Rhondi and David Anderson about the cost effectiveness of birth in America.

Corrupting Factor of Health Care

In many ways the fact that so much money rides on women bearing children has corrupted the way birth is handled. Instead of medicine as a ministry to people, altruistic and patient centered, the industry has become a very big "big business" out to make a profit. Instead of providing evidence-based care, doctors provide birth services that support the bottom line. When a woman births in a hospital, several financial factors are in play. First, there is a breakeven point on how long a woman can stay in the hospital before the hospital loses money. After so many hours, the birth becomes less and less financially profitable. The staff has to be paid, the bed basically rented, etc. Hospitals have to pay for all those expensive furnishing, medical machines, and 24-hour round the clock staffing. Then there are insurance issues – most of medical care is paid for through medical insurance. We shouldn't be surprised that women who have good private insurance have more interventional procedures than those with public assistance like Medicare. The more the insurance pays for, the more of these services are used and billed. Hospitals cannot survive without billing insurance.

Another corruption in the medical community is how new technologies and medications are evaluated. Instead of having non-biased objective research, the manufacturers publish their own finding – how can these not be biased? No systematic evaluation process exists for new medical equipment. Yet since the equipment is developed so quickly, and so much money rides on it sale, the new technologies are aggressively promoted to physicians. The industry continues developing new high-cost technologies, marketing them to hospitals and doctors. They give free samples of drugs; they take the doctors out to lunch or bring them food at their offices. Doctors buy into the marketing even if the equipment or drugs haven't been studied effectively. This is a huge multi-billion dollar part of the U.S. economy. Things like the Electronic Fetal Monitor, which costs ten to twenty thousand dollars, have never been proven in scientific studies to improve the mortality of women or their babies. The industry doesn't even have standards for the electrical output of the machine? The machines do not have to hold to any standards of engineering as well. Medicine should be based on science not on good sales pitches and commercial bribery.

But, it's all about the money. The technology industry encourages the equipment's use regardless as to its ability to help people. So it is market and economic issues that bring about much of what is done in health care rather than what is in the best interests of the public. Equipment, though high in cost, is favored instead of using human touch. The cost of health care technology is one of the reasons for the rapid increase in insurance costs. The healthcare industry uses this equipment because they are sold on technology like most of the rest of North Americans.

Convenience Rules

Most alarming are the unscientific procedures and protocols that doctors use in the hospitals. Everything is geared on the turnaround time of a birth. A hospital only makes money on a birth if it occurs within a certain time period. Much of what doctors do is to keep their patients on schedule. They call it active management. Statistics bear out the fact that the majority of hospital births occur between 9 am and 5 pm, Monday through Friday. When women fail to progress in early labor, instead of being sent home, they are given strong medicines to hurry labor along, though these medications can bring about serious and deadly complications. Many times one complication leads to another. Once a woman steps into a hospital, she is on the timetable of the birth machine. Doctor's have appointments to make during their office hours. They may also have several other women all birthing at the same time. They can't afford to sit with a woman through a long labor. Some doctors are using multimedia systems that allow them to check in with a birthing woman while they are still in their offices seeing the rest of their patients. This saves them from canceling any appointments until the last minute.

Obstetrics is always trying to speed up birth or to make it more convenient and controlled. For instance powerful drugs used in managing labor are often studied for effectiveness, but not for efficacy – this means their safety isn't a factor. Doctors use some medications that have been reported to increase the risk for babies and mothers. The doctors will even use medications to induce labor that are not approved by the FDA (Federal Drug Administration) for obstetrical purposes.

Avoiding Lawsuits

Another reason obstetricians push for interventions is that they are afraid of being sued in courts and having their malpractice insurance rates increase. Seventy percent of obstetricians have been sued (Ryan 1988) – obstetricians have the highest amount of lawsuits each year compared with other medical service providers. These doctors routinely use an electronic fetal monitor without any medical justification, but it is obvious that they feel protected by having the machine since it provides a tangible piece of evidence if anything does go wrong – the strip the machine prints out is used as evidence in court. However there is documented proof that electronic fetal monitoring does not improve fetal outcomes or offer any benefit to the mother, and it is prone to high false readings and failings. Therefore the routine use of electronic fetal monitors exposes obstetricians to greater liability. The simple intermittent auscultation of the fetal heart rate provides equal if not better information than the EFM and can offer physicians more protection from liability when auscultation is utilized as the standard of care (Lent 1999).

Another way doctors try to avoid legal complications is to perform c-sections. A cesarean may be performed even when there is no medical reason – some people plan to have their children this way. Many doctors feel legally protected about birth if they can perform this surgery; this is defensive medicine. The fundamental part of the Hippocratic Oath is to primarily do what is in the benefit of the patient not the doctor. But greed and fear make a dangerous mix.

The United States has over 35,000 obstetricians and about 5,000 midwives. Great Britain has 32,000 Midwives and 1,000 Obstetricians. Britain has less than an 8% cesarean rate and the US has more than 30%. 50 to 80 percent of births in the U.S. involve some surgical procedure; remember obstetricians are highly trained surgeons – that's what they learned how to do, and that's how they make the most money. So you can understand why a surgical birth is easier for a doctor. For one it gives them almost complete control. Secondly, it also pays them the highest amount. Thirdly it is on their schedule. And, fourthly, a cesarean has less chance in their eyes of causing litigation.

Midwives

There are very few midwives in the U.S. The doctors in this country have effectively eliminated midwifery for about one hundred years. There was a concerted effort by doctors between 1900 and 1930 to eliminate their competition. Dr. Kloosterman, renowned Chief of Obstetrics and Gynecology at the University of Amsterdam, Holland, states "All over the world there exists in every society a small group of women who feel themselves strongly attracted to giving care to other women during pregnancy and childbirth. Failure to make use of this group of highly motivated people is regrettable and a sin" *against the whole of society* (our emphasis).

Out of the 5,000 midwives in the country, most are nurse midwives who are under the authority of medical doctors at the hospitals where they work. Midwives reduce the cost of birth, and their numbers of birth per year has continuously increased. In 1999, 7.7 percent of hospital births were in their hands. Most freestanding birth centers are in the hands of midwives as well. Usually the midwives have less restraint from the medical establishment in such a center, so they are able to provide a more holistic style of childbirth services.

In many progressive states, direct entry midwifery is becoming legal again. These states require midwives to go through a licensing process. However, though midwives are increasing in numbers and have better outcomes by far, they still find extreme prejudice in North American society. Though doctor's and midwives both lose babies – meaning that even the best of care cannot stop neonatal or postnatal deaths, but only the midwives are persecuted in criminal courts. Midwives have been interviewed on television news shows when they have lost a child. All people view the death of a newborn as tragic, so this type of publicity can destroy a midwife's career. Unfortunately, it is the societal belief that modern medicine is superior that causes the stigma for midwives. We know that there has been a smear campaign against midwives for over 100 years. Despite all this negativity, midwives still practice and provide superior care for low risk pregnancies.

The legal issues have been the greatest barriers for midwifery's revival in North America. Midwives before licensing practiced under threat of criminal prosecution – many still do. Some midwives fortunately were radicals and feminists who believed in improving women's healthcare at any cost and who faced the patriarchal medical industry, defying its laws and rhetoric. Many midwives being trained today either in direct entry relationships or through nurse-midwifery programs are influenced by these strong-willed women. Birth to a great deal of women is a woman's political issue. Almost no men become midwives, but most doctors are men. Even the women doctors who are trained in the male dominated medical field are apt to practice obstetrics like their male counterparts. Often these women have never had children themselves. Regardless of their lengthy and expensive training, most obstetricians have never sat through a full natural childbirth.

Midwives work in all the states, but the protection under the law is still at issue. Midwives Alliance of North America (MANA) maintains a state to state listing, including the District of Columbia listing of the current legal status of midwifery. You can check on your states status by going to MANA's home page http://mana.org/links.html.

Cost of Birth

What is birth going to cost? You may not care, but the insurance you may have may only offer you certain choices, so you really need to know if you are covered, especially if you choose an alternative type of birth. In the Journal of Nurse-Midwifery, Vol. 44, No. 1, January/February 1999, an article written by Rhondi and David Anderson, compares three types of births. Accordingly, the average uncomplicated vaginal birth costs 68% less in a home than in a hospital, while births initiated in the home offer a lower combined rate of intrapartum and neonatal mortality and a lower incidence of cesarean delivery.

In 1998, the general charge for home births was $1,823 (the high being about $4,500 and the low $800 nationally. The Health Insurance Association of America reports that the average total charge for uncomplicated vaginal deliveries [in hospitals] at the same time was $7,567 and in birth centers the cost would be around $4,050. Based on the data from 1998, the average home birth for an uncomplicated vaginal birth was 24% of a hospital birth and 45% of a birth center birth. These figures do not take into account the enormous differences in the cost of living geographically since they are all averages. This means that a home delivery saves an estimated 76% from birth in the hospital and 55% of a birth center.

Hospital costs are much higher due to the hospital fees that average 55% of these charges. An additional average cost of $4,331 can be added for a cesarean section, bringing the total cost to $11,898. Since childbirth makes up one-fifth of all health care expenditures and is the most frequent cause for hospital admission, you can see that the medical establishment needs births financially.

The total amount of births according to the U.S. Department of Health and Human Services in 1999 was just under 4 million (just over in 2002), you can see that the economics of birth are huge. 7.7 percent of these births occurred with midwives. That leaves a meager 1% outside the hospital, divided between freestanding birth centers (27%) and midwives (65%) with the remainder probably either planned or unplanned home births.

That means 3,960,000 births occurred in hospitals. 871,200 women delivered surgically at a total charge of $10,365,537,600. The rest brought in $29,965,320,000. Birth represents $40,330,857,600.

Birth center births worked with approximately 10,800 births at $4050, coming to $43,740,000. While another 16,900 births were midwife-attended at home at $1,823 a piece, coming to $30,808,700. That means that all 5,000 midwives are responsible for only 8.3% of birth in this country. In most nations in Europe, midwives handle 75% or more of births are handled. Obstetricians handle the rest. The midwives handle the normal births, while the doctors handle the difficult and problematic births.

According to an article in Health Day Newsby Robert Preidt the stats continue to grow:

The total number of births rose to 4,317,119 in 2007, the highest number of births ever registered in the United States. The Cesarean delivery rate increased by 2 percent to 31.8 percent in 2007.

Current estimates are bantered about. The most recent estimated value of childbirth in the US has risen to 86 billion dollars, while the costs have more than doubled since 1999.

The Economic Pie

Birth represents the most important chunk of the economic pie of the medical establishment. That is assuredly the main reason why malpractice insurance is extremely difficult or impossible for midwives and birth centers to obtain. Without coverage, midwives and birth centers are under the whole risk of birth, and since babies die occasional regardless of the care received, they are staking their personal livelihood and possibly their family's to serve the families they work with. Medical doctors control these malpractice insurance companies, so by denying midwives access to insurance they can hamstring or reduce their competition. In the United States the cost of health insurance continues to rise. Safe and inexpensive alternatives are available, and as the statistics bear out, more and more women are choosing to birth with midwives. According to the research the Anderson's presented, there is no question that midwifery services are both safer and more cost effective. Because of these social and economic issues, many HMO's are staffing their maternity wards with midwives.

Paying for the Birth

When we had our four children, we began learning about the cost of birth for us fathers. For our first child's birth we had an extremely good insurance package, and it covered all but $16 for parking. Genny had premature labor and was put on bed rest, so she was a prime candidate for receiving care from the obstetricians. The total cost for that birth in 1988 was around $20,000. When our last child was born, we paid for a home birth with a midwife. The cost was $2,000 cash. We would pay the midwife $200 each prenatal visit. The first birth was a scary, stressful and complicated birth requiring surgery – well before we knew anything much about birth, so we were very thankful for the medical care and the good healthcare insurance. Then when we had the home birth, we felt the investment was well worth it because our son's birth was simple and serene.

The issue here is a big one for us guys. We often pay for these births either through our insurance or from our checking accounts. If you are self employed and pay for insurance you may have to add a rider to your policy to cover childbirth at all. These days childbirth can be very expensive so think about the bottom line. Depending on what type of insurance you have or don't have, you need to learn what options you have. What providers are covered and which ones aren't. Without insurance, how will you finance the birth? We've made the following table to give you some ideas (all averages). These prices change as the medical and birth fields inflate their costs due to economic and demographic changes.

Non-surgical Birth

	Cost for Home Birth with Midwife	Cost of Freestanding Birth Center	Cost of Nurse Midwife in Hospital	Cost for Doctor
No Insurance	$1,800	$4,050	$7,567	$7,567
Insurance	$1,800	Check coverage	Check coverage	0

Emergency Surgical Birth

	Cost for Home Birth with Midwife	Cost of Freestanding Birth Center	Cost of Nurse Midwife in Hospital	Cost for Doctor
No Insurance	$1,800* + Hospital Approximately $3,500 Emergency Transport $600 Total $5,900	$4,050* + Hospital Approximately $3,500 Emergency Transport $600 Total $8,150	$11,898	$11,898
Insurance	$1,800	Check coverage	Check coverage	0**

*   Transfer to hospital
**   There may be co-pays or deductibles.

For fun look at the following internet link to see what the cost use to be for birth:

http://journeytocrunchville.wordpress.com/2008/08/04/flashback-cost-of-birth-in-america-in-1957/

Remember only if you have a low risk pregnancy will most certified professional midwives take your partner's care. If you want a birth center birth, you may have to advocate for that with your insurance company. If you prefer midwives in the hospital, you need to check to see if your coverage covers them. Many insurance plans only cover a set group of providers, so this may limit your ability to choose. Doctors are always covered, but sometimes only partially depending on what your insurance dictates as far as primary care physicians, etc. Then there are deductibles. When we had our first birth, we had no deductibles to pay. You may also have a co-pay for prenatal and post partum visits. If you chose to pay for a home or birth center birth, you will see that if an emergency occurs, your insurance should cover you unless there are stipulations on with whom or where medical services must occur. Transfers occur in about 8% of home births. We hope this helps you understand the basics of how to cover the cost of your birth.

Changes in American Insurance

Since the previous research was reported, health insurance has continued to rise in cost. New health plans are being offered to Americans that they pay themselves. This is changing the way families are facing the rising cost of birth. Today it is reported that an average uncomplicated birth costs $14,000 in total.

Todd Zwillich from WebMD Health News reported in the summer of 2007 in an article titled: Childbirth and Pregnancy Often Uncovered in Plans, that most so-called "consumer-directed" health plans do not cover maternity costs. 60% of Americans are covered by employer's insurance which does cover childbirth expenses. But with these new insurance plans for those who are stuck with limited options, this can be critical. Also as health care costs escalate, many insurance plans have raised their deductibles. Pregnancy can force you to pay two year's of deductibles as many pregnancies cover two years – starting in one year and ending in another. He adds further:

> Assuming an uncomplicated pregnancy ending in a vaginal birth, patients would pay between $1,455 and $7,884 out-of-pocket, depending on how generous the consumer-directed plan. But a complicated birth requiring a cesarean section, early labor, or a newborn stay in a neonatal intensive care can balloon out-of-pocket costs to $8,800 for the most generous plan and a staggering $21,200 for the least generous.

These consumer-directed plans often require expensive riders to cover childbirth and pregnancy. They often require high deductibles of $5,000 per person or $10,000 per family. Childbirth can often bring the expenses out of pocket to these levels, so that would mean you would pay these costs yourself.

Consumer Driven Change Warranted

As with most enterprises, when consumers are not getting what they want, there is a backlash of negative consumer feedback. Organizations have been founded to address the over use of surgery and interventions. Even Consumer Reports states on their website: "Despite growing evidence of harm, many obstetricians and maternity hospitals still overuse high-tech procedures that can mean poorer outcomes for baby and Mom." This statement was followed by a quiz they prepared. You can see it at the following web address:

http://www.consumerreports.org/health/medical-conditions-treatments/pregnancy-childbirth/maternity-care/maternity-care-quiz/maternity-care-quiz.htm

This shows how relevant the issues are with consumers for this popular magazine to include childbirth in their consumer issues. These issues are ripe for social movements to improve maternity health care.

Chapter 15: Advocating for Alternatives

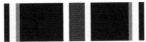

If you choose to find alternatives to the normal way birth is handled in North America, you will find it requires effort, perseverance, fortitude, and other investments of your time and/or money. Advocacy generally requires a great deal from you, so you had better be motivated. You and your partner are the consumers, and you should have a say in your care. You are paying, or your insurance provider is paying, a great deal of money, for the birth. They as well as you have a right for cost effective and safe services. If you approach your insurance company with data, you may even be able to broaden your choice options.

Finding A Doctor With An Alternative Philosophy

If you want an alternative to a hospital birth, you may be inclined to just look for doctor with an alternative or more holistic philosophy. Also make sure that theme permeates the medical practices of the doctor's partners or you may end up facing an unwanted type of service. Many times a liberal-minded doctor is on the fringe of the medical profession and other doctors will not work with him or her, so they may hide their philosophical bent. Don't be deceived. Know what the practice you associate with is like and what each individual doctor is like. Remember many of these doctors and as a matter of fact the nurses who espouse alternative philosophies are taking risks for your care.

Finding a doctor with a track record of lower episiotomies, cesarean sections and other interventions requires research. Interviews take time and effort. Getting this all done may be well worth your time however, so don't be disheartened. Pregnancy takes a while and so does finding the right doctor and hospital for your birth. You should count yourself lucky if you find a private practice that will discuss their statistics with you, the consumer, at all.

Alternative Birthing Room

We have already discussed how birthing rooms were cosmetically changed as a result of consumer demands back in the eighties. These rooms are still in operation, but doctors still practice their brand of medicine and use every intervention possible regardless of the veneer on the door. An alternative birthing room is not an alternative birth unless the staff has alternative thinking. The fact that you are in the environment of the medical establishment really means you are under their jurisdiction. However, your insurance will readily pay for this type of alternative.

Midwives in the Hospital

We've read a great deal regarding the level of intervention of midwives versus doctors in the hospital. It appears that midwives who practice in the hospital are much less likely to use interventions than doctors. Their stats are a big improvement. Many HMO's even use midwives to lower the cost of birth in hospitals.

Their rights to practice in a hospital are usually completely controlled by doctors as well. But since you are looking for an option covered by your insurance, this may be the easiest alternative to obtain. Just ask the midwives questions that will bring out their philosophical bent. Interview the midwife just as you would interview a physician or any other health care provider. You may find some midwives practice just like doctors, using as many interventions. Others may be more focused on natural childbirth, using few interventions. You will know after an interview or two.

Taking a Caregiver with You

Going into the birth machine with a mature and experience advocate may be another option you try. Labor assistants or Doulas can do what nurses are constrained from doing these days and that is advocate for your partner's rights. You may feel confidant yourself in handling this, but many men just feel inadequate with dealing with health issues. However, it may be in your best interests, especially if you are avoiding unnecessary interventions, to hire someone who really knows the birth machine's tactics. Costs range from $500 to $1200 for an able person. So, if you can't find a doctor who agrees with you and your partner's desires for a natural birth, bring someone with you to your prenatal appointments and birth. It's your health care dollar, and the cost of a Doula or labor assistant is an additional charge. An advocate may cost monetarily, but evading a surgery is priceless.

Freestanding Birth Centers

Further from the central core of a technocratic birth, you may find you have the option of using a freestanding birth center. Some insurance policies allow payment to these facilities. We have in our own time had to write and convince Blue Cross to pay for using one, demonstrating the cost savings and to justify the safety. This is still cutting edge for many medical insurance providers today. If the medical community owns the birth center, than it is obviously going to guarantee that insurance will cover it. But many birth centers are owned and operated by a group of professional midwives. Since they are on the fringe of the medical community, and, since insurance carriers are often managed by medical doctors (just like malpractice insurance), it is difficult for them to get their services approved. That means their services may have to be funded directly out of your pocket.

For birth centers to become accredited requires a huge and professional effort. So these places are very serious about setting up business and require a big investment of those running them. The statistics for these centers are excellent. That is one of the reasons people are willing to pay the expenses out of pocket.

The problem with birth centers is that there aren't enough to go around. The 200 or so in North America cannot possible cover the need. However, in the past, before midwives were legal again, the more adventuresome would fly to an area with a birth center, and take a vacation until their baby came. Some doctors who had a very alternative type of practice also would have similar stories to share of couples flying down from other states to birth with them.

Home Birth: The Art of Midwifery

Home birth is most likely a new type of service to be paid for by your insurance carrier. They may not have handled this request before, but since midwives are professional service providers, who are licensed by states, they can be covered if you ask. Because you have x number of dollars provided for in your insurance package for maternity care, you should be able to apply it to an alternative type of service provider. It wasn't too many years ago that acupuncture and chiropractic care were not covered and now they are on many insurance plans. Home birth is likely to be standardized in the future. Yet since less than 1% of births are done in the home, most insurance companies have not seen this type of request before.

The risk of birthing at home is that no one is giving midwives proper liability insurance. This means that you and your partner must take on the responsibility of your birth. Remember it has only been for a few years since midwives have won the right to offer services legally, and in some states they still cannot practice legally. Many of the midwives working in the United States have been arrested for practicing medicine.

Midwives are the most apt to let your partner birth the way she wants. This requires little interference from you. This means your partner is going to have much more control over how she births. Another positive is that the cost is only 22% on average of a hospital birth. The downside is that most insurance companies will only cover state licensed practitioners – that means your cost may be the whole charge if your insurance will not pay. Since there are only a few midwives in most communities, you will have a smaller group of professionals to choose from. In Orange County, California, you may only find a handful of midwives servicing a population of 2 million plus. Outlying areas often have more midwives to go around. However, remember it is the holistic philosophy that most people are paying for. The lower rate of intervention and the better odds of having a healthy baby are often a worthwhile option.

Midwifery is Not the Practice of Medicine

Midwifery is not the practice of medicine. The definition of the practice of medicine seems to pivot around drugs and medicines. A common definition for the practice of medicine is the treatment of diseases or accidents with medicine or drugs. The key to the definition of midwifery is the condition of normalcy. At its most simple definition midwifery is the art and science of caring for women undergoing normal pregnancies, and the providing of assistance to a woman during a normal course of labor and childbirth. Pregnancy and birth are normal physiological processes. Pregnancy is not a disease nor is birth an accident. The art of midwifery is unique and is something else from the practice of medicine or nursing. The World Health Organization adds "that, because midwifery and nursing are separate disciplines, they should be studied, considered, and regulated separately." For those interested in a greater understanding of how midwifery is not the practice of medicine, and more information on the subject. We highly recommend *Midwifery is Not the Practice of Medicine* a journal article by Suzanne Hope Suarez RN, BSN, J.D... This definitive treatise on the subject originally was published in the Yale Journal of Law and Feminism, and is supported by over three hundred references.

Getting Insurance Carriers to Pay

Most insurance carriers will give ear to a cost savings for medical services. That is the best way to approach them. They know the average cost of medical services of hospitals and are always looking to reduce those costs. So if you prefer alternative birth locations or alternative caregivers, you may have to write some letters to your human resources staff benefits office; ask them for the name of the account representative for your insurance provider. Then you can contact and tell them what you would like to do. Even midwives who assist your partner to birth in your own home can be covered if you can get through to the insurance provider. Some providers, especially HMO's with their own maternity wards and hospitals generally will not cover independent care providers for your birth, but other private insurance may be more flexible. HMO's sometimes staff their hospital labor and delivery with midwives, so you may have an alternative readily available. Write your insurance company to learn of the current options available to you.

We went through this process to get insurance to pay for a birth center birth in Indianapolis. Phil began by writing staff benefits. He began at the bottom, writing first the person responsible for the policy. Later he wrote his boss; each time he detailed how the birth center would give Genny the type of birth she wanted and would save the insurance company money. The decision is always in the hands of the staff benefits people. It is your employer's decision; they may try to put it off on the insurance company, but the control of the decision on who gets covered is in the hands of your staff benefits people. They told Phil then that it would have to be Blue Cross that okayed a birth center, but Blue Cross continuously denied that saying it just required authorization from staff benefits.

After talking with the director of Blue Cross of Indiana, we still got nowhere. Phil ended up writing the director of staff benefits and telling him that the insurance provider expressly said that they had the ability to authorize the use of this alternative birth facility. This was 1993. At the time Blue Cross national had only covered one other birth center birth up in New York State.

Alternative care providers, like midwives, will already know more than we do regarding which insurance providers will cover them. You might call some as soon as you are aware that your partner is pregnant, if you chose alternative types of service. In approaching an insurance company about provision for an alternative modality of care it is important to remember the power phrases that you are not asking your insurer for something new or a new benefit, You are asking for care that is cost effective for them and that is satisfying for the consumer. This all should be taken care of as soon as possible. The more quickly you two have done your research and prepared your written requests the better, for you will have laid out the two most important parts of your mission which is choosing the care provider and the location of the birth.

Top Brass

As in many situations, if you give your responsibility and authority to another party, you are giving your rights away. Birth services like any other services are yours for the choosing. You are the consumer, and it is your dollar (or your insurance dollar) paying for the services. If men would stand up and begin protecting their women from the birth machine, from incompetent practices, and from bureaucratic policy, then the way birth is handled in the country would change. By demanding that insurance carriers pay for alternative care, you exercise your authority. When a whole group of men do this, then we as a group can make a difference.

Besides pressuring the insurance carriers, you should know the birth is just one of many women's health issues being debated in national legislatures. States and provinces also discuss these important topics. If in your area midwifery is still illegal, then you should write your legislative representation and ensure women's reproductive health issues are addressed, including the provision of midwifery care. Do not let the birth machine and its big bucks scare you. People have authority in a democratic society. The more voices demanding change, the more impetus to change.

Men have stood by too long letting the medical establishment control and dominant birth. In the seventies, men started getting more involved with birth. A few bold men stepped across the threshold and stood by their mates in the labor and delivery rooms. They took childbirth classes. They got involved with coaching birth. Yet as long as men handed their wives and partners off to the doctor's authority, they got the same results. Now it is time for men across North America to say "No More" to western medicine's harsh handling of birth. Why should we as a whole pay the highest in the world for childbirth services, yet receive the 28th best care? Why should we have a 31.8 percent cesarean rate when most of the best countries have rates of less than ten percent? The best countries in the world for mortality rates still have the vast majority of babies with midwives; so why shouldn't we?

Women have been trying to make these changes for years. They may think that they can generate enough political and social power to handle this on their own, but we know this world is still dominated by men. When was the last time a woman was elected President of the United States though Hilliary Clinton made it look possible? We as men have the power to make this change, but it isn't going to happen without us each individually taking charge. We've got to take on the medical policies; we've got to stop the intrusive interventions. Each of us needs to demand that birth happens the way our partner's want, rather than giving them over to a machine that chews up our women and spits them and our babies out.

Real men take the responsibility for the birth of their children. So as you step forward to protect your partner and your baby and as you make the calls and write the letters, you force the issue of safer childbirth. You advocate for a better and saner world when you become politically involved with this issue. You are the top brass, so go and exercise your authority. Let's change things. Childbirth is not meant to be a violation of women.

Remember the greatest way to make these changes is find out what your partner wants, and ensuring she has a choice in who she births with, where she births, and the policies governing that birth environment. The more people demand their rights to choice as consumers, the more force this type of movement will have.

Chapter 16: Dealing with the Unexpected

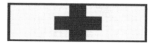

Flying the mission, you need not be overly concerned about complications. You should expect that things will go well – the odds are in your favor. Know that your inexperience can cause you to view variations of birth as overly serious, so that is why you hire an experienced attendant to determine if anything major is happening. Since complications do occur in a small percentage of pregnancies and childbirth, you need to face the unknown. Should anything happen, you need to be informed; this will help you and your partner make better decisions under fire. First there are three types of complications to look at. There are those that need immediate resolution. Then there are those demanding immediate attention. Then there are those, which require evaluation.

Think of them in terms of alert status. The first are emergency situations. The second could lead to emergency status if not taken care of. The third are more like long-term concerns. As long as you understand the complications and how to deal with them, you eliminate the fear and the anxiety regarding birth.

Flares Up Early

Your partner may have medical conditions that immediately send up flares that pregnancy and childbirth may be difficult. These issues are usually scored "High Risk." Should your partner have any of the following conditions, you should seek expert medical care for that condition, to ensure the pregnancy doesn't cause health issues.

- Twins or more
- Pre-eclampsia
- High blood pressure
- Weak or scarred Cervix
- 3 or more miscarriages
- Growth retardation
- Genetic disorders
- Seizure disorders

- Gross Overweight
- Gross Underweight
- Disease
- Diabetes
- Heart Disease
- Over 35
- Early pregnancy bleeding
- Previous surgery to reproductive organs

With these conditions, pregnancy can cause your partner's body additional stress, and therefore more caution should be observed. For more significant illnesses, the developing baby is at higher risk as well. Studies show that the risk of having a stillborn child is higher if a woman has an infection early on in pregnancy, even if it is treated with antibiotics. So if a woman has other physical problems with her body before becoming pregnant, the risks involved are evident. Because these situations are known before the birth, your partner's pregnancy may be labeled "High Risk."

When Your Partner Needs the Medic

When your partner is healthy, the odds are in your favor. You should be happy. But any trained pilot learns the ejection procedures. You need to be able to recognize when things are getting out of hand. You should know when the baby or your partner is in trouble. Of course, we suggest that you have a professional working with you to give you and your partner advice. Knowledge is empowering, so just put these things in the back of your mind in case. When and if pregnancy or labor ceases to be within the scope of normalcy it is time for a consultation with or the transfer of care to an obstetrician. Where midwifery's forte is normal pregnancy and childbirth obstetrics is the art and medical science of caring for abnormal pregnancies, labors and births.

Shock

Your partner may go into shock. Shock can occur during or after a birth. Shock if not treated can lead to death. The likelihood is low, but you should be able to recognize if your partner is going into shock. Symptoms include rapid pulse rate (over 90 beats per minute), sweaty or clammy skin and an abnormal breathing pattern (deep and then shallow). Your partner may become disoriented and have poor reflexes as well. Shock is usually associated with hemorrhaging – sometimes not noticed due to the placenta blocking external blood flow. Shock can also occur from some other internal bleeding or from dehydration or exhaustion.

If in shock, your partner, if not in the hospital, should be transported ASAP. Generally this is a medically justified reason for a cesarean section. When someone goes into shock, they should put their feet up while lying down (keeping the blood in the cranium); they should be covered in a blanket to keep warm; and they should be given fluids. Transport to the hospital is necessary for home or birth center birth.

Excessive Bleeding During Birth

Bleeding occurs because the placenta is connected to the uterus, and must detach. If the bleeding occurs before the birth, this could mean the placenta is detaching too early. That is critical because the baby must breathe through the umbilical cord, and that cord gets its oxygen from the placenta. The medical term for this complication is abrupio placenta (placenta pulls away from uterus before birth).

All women have some bleeding. At the onset of labor there is the loss of the mucus plug, sometimes even called the bloody show. At the beginning of pregnancy the opening to the cervix fills with mucus this is what is known as the mucus plug. As the cervix ripens and effaces the mucus plug is released and a red or pinky watery spot of mucus is let go from the cervix. All through the course of labor as the baby's head presses against the cervix and as the cervix opens up there may be small amounts of blood visible. Any time your care provider is concerned with the quality or amount of blood loss at a birth it is important to transfer care, a woman can only lose so much blood before it becomes an emergency.

Cardic Arrest

This almost never happens unless drugs are involved or the woman has a known heart condition or defect. Drugs that drop the blood pressure can prove fatal. Epidurals and cytotec are known to drop blood pressure. Knowing what drugs drop blood pressure should help you to avoid this danger.

Respiration

Another problem that can occur is that your partner may stop breathing. Again this is more often associated with medications interfering with the nervous system or the numbing of the diaphragm. Without medications you should have nothing to worry about.

Postpartum Hemorrhage

Postpartum hemorrhage occurs mostly in hospital birth but happens occasionally at home or at a birth center. The following are causes: Use of pitocin for inductions and labor enhancing, midforceps delivery, forceps rotation, incisions in the uterus or cervix, uterine atony due to anesthesia, too much haste in removing a placenta, too early cutting of the umbilical cord, and manual removal of the placenta (which can take up to an hour in some case naturally). Cigarette smokers have the worst time with this issue.

When Your Baby Needs the Medic

Several complications can affect the baby's health during a birth. Several exist after a birth. There are times when babies need serious attention.

Unfortunately not all babies are going to make it. The chances of a baby surviving before 24 weeks gestational age are almost zero – though it does happen. Babies are supposed to be born between 38 to 40 weeks some later. Some babies haven't developed properly and others have congenital defects that make living outside of the womb impossible. These factors are not something you control. If your partner goes into premature labor before 36 weeks, then you should realize if the baby is born, it might need serious medical attention. Now, for the vast majority of births, the birth occurs between 36 and 42 weeks gestation. The complications you need to know about follow.

Fetal Heart Rates

First while the birth is going on, your care provider will be checking the heart rate of the baby. Everything about the baby's safety is related to keeping a consistent 120 to 160 beats per minute. Professionals generally use a fetoscope or a Doppler for checking these rates. Rates are generally checked every half an hour in first stage, and every fifteen minutes during transition, then every ten minutes during second stage.

When a baby's heart rates run below or above average (below 100, or over 180) then the baby may be showing signs of distress. If the baby has a high rate, it usually is because the baby isn't getting enough oxygen so the heart pumps faster. If lower, then possibly the baby's heart itself isn't getting enough oxygen to pump the blood adequately. Either way fetal distress can signify serious complications for the baby.

Changing a mother's position can sometimes relieve the fetal distress especially if the cord is being pinched between the baby's head and the uterine wall. The on-all-fours position can sometimes loosen the cord. Having your partner lie on her left side can also help improve the amount of circulation to the placenta.

Fetal distress can come about due to medications that speed up a slow-going labor. Many of the cesarean sections performed in North American institutions are because of this condition. The four main reasons for this surgical procedure include fetal distress, dystocia (baby gets stuck), repeat cesarean, and breech presentation.

Prolapsed Cord

We have discussed how to avoid a prolapsed cord, but you should know what needs to be done in case one occurs. The cord in this position means the uterus is going to cut off the oxygen flow through the cord, and that spells trouble for the baby. This can happen when the bag of waters breaks since the surge of water can push the cord down, trapping it between the baby's head and the uterine wall, or possible pushing it through the cervix and into the vagina. If this occurs during the first stage of the labor, then you should be headed for a medically necessary cesarean section.

Apgar Score

A doctor named Virgina Apgar developed a scale that rates the level of health of a baby after birth. If your baby is born with a low score, you may have a medical emergency. This is especially true if, after the baby is born, it is pale or blue and limp or without movement.

Sign	0	1	2
Heart Rate	Absent	Below 100 beats per minute	Above 100 beats per minute
Respiratory Effort	Absent	Slow or irregular	Good and strong
Muscle Tone	Limp	Some flexion of extremities	Active Motion
Reflex irritability to lips being touch	No Response	Grimace	Couch, sneeze or strong grimace
Skin Color	Blue	Partially pink, but blue at extremities	Pink all over

The scale tells the tale. Should your baby need resuscitation, your care provider should be on top of it. Warrant any caregiver you hire can handle resuscitation. It only takes a few minutes without air after the birth before a baby succumbs.

Attention

These concerns require attention, but do not necessarily lead to emergencies. They are signs that things are difficult.

<u>Partner's Not Handling Contractions</u>

There are a few reasons exist for why your partner may not be handling her contractions well. One simply may be dehydration or lack of certain electrolytes. This is more frequent in long hard labors where the woman has worked hard and depleted her reserve. In many ways birth is like a marathon, or other events of physical endurance. You may have participated in an event like "triple overtime" and know exhaustion personally so you can empathize. Your care provider should have a protocol in place for replacing lost fluids. You can encourage your partner to drink or take sips after every contraction.

Sometimes the laboring woman may need a change of scenery, position or environment. Someone may be present who is detracting from the labor or the mother may need the presence of someone there who is not. She simply may need to be left alone or to get in the shower. Explore all options. The sense of losing control over contractions in itself is almost a natural process of giving birth, and her losing control may not mean anything more than the labor is transitioning from opening up the cervix to prepare for the pushing out of the baby. Transition is often the shortest of the phases of labor but is the most intense. If the woman is in transition, it is helpful to reassure her that it won't be long and that her body is doing exactly what it is suppose to do. Frequently after transition there is a natural pause in labor that may be designed to allow the mother to regroup and rest between contractions before she actively begins pushing.

A hard labor is like running up mountains. When you run short of breathe and energy, you become disoriented and start feeling you are losing it. If this is occurring just before the second stage of labor, some women can pull through, but if it is earlier on in early or active labor, interventions might just offer relief. If she continues voicing panic and fear, touch base with your care provider and see if it is best to get medical attention. Often times the health care provider may understand the territory of birth and can help you and your partner navigate through its course. The care provider should have a whole load of tricks packed with them to help a woman get back on top of her labor. However sometimes, and for some women, it is necessary for them to receive a small dosage of a medication to cut the intensity of the contractions to help her to recuperate and to be able to handle the contractions.

Meconium Staining

Meconium is the greenish black substance within the baby's intestinal tract that makes for his first bowel movement. Bill Cosby most noticeably references this as being the combination of Velcro and tar. When a baby passes a bowel movement before the birth it stains the amniotic fluids and is known as meconium staining. This occurs in approximately 12% of all births (Ross 2005). It is considered to be a low risk obstetrical hazard. The presence of meconium in the amniotic fluid complicates things but does not have to derail the course of labor and birth. The concern is to prevent the baby from breathing in meconium at the time of its birth, a condition known as meconium aspiration syndrome. The management of meconium staining is all determined by the degree of its presence. The meconium may be delectated by an amnion infusion in the hospital before birth, or steps can be taken to be proactive in preventing the baby from inhaling the meconium as he is born. There are certain degrees and consistencies of meconium that will call for more aggressive management of the labor and birth.

Precipitous (Fast) Labor

Some women birth their babies fast. Their contractions are almost magnified, without any enhancement from anything else. Precipitous labor is an active labor shorter than three hours. Some ladies give birth within two hours of the first contraction. It is not known for certain how many women experience precipitous labor. One author records 2% as the percent of labors occurring precipitously (Ventura 1995). The whole affair is stressful because the uterus is working extra fast and hard. Now when the contractions are coming hard and fast, this can cause fetal distress. The possibility of hemorrhaging increases. There is a greater likelihood of soft tissue tears because the birth is occurring so quickly these tissues are not given the opportunity to gradually stretch. The baby's head may receive some trauma as it quickly passes through the bony pelvis. All in all, however, a precipitous labor demonstrates how well the body is coordinating for the efficient birth of the baby. A birth for the mother without having the opportunity to rest between contractions is a stressful ordeal, so she may need to distress about this after the birth. Listen to her and emphasize with her regarding this momentous birth.

Cord Around the Baby's Neck, Back , and Shoulder

In about half of all births the cord will be wrapped around the baby in some way, either the shoulder and back or the neck. When the cord is wrapped around the neck, it is called a nuchal cord. This happens 25% of the time, and is not often a serious complication. Genny remarks that when she works with midwives and a baby is presented for delivery with the cord over the shoulder or around the back, it would be mused that the baby was coming packing a back pack too!

The danger has to do with pulling on the cord and disrupting the placenta before it is detaching. The baby is still breathing through the cord, even after it is out, you will see it pulsing. Some people chose not to cut the cord until the pulsing stops. Your care provider should be able to easily loop the cord off a baby's neck. If the cord is so tight around the neck that your care provider can't get it off, then they may clamp and cut the cord before the birth. When this happens, the baby must be born without delay.

Variable Presentation

Babies are born all the time in a breech position. About 39% of breech babies are born in the hospital by cesarean section. Some women will find all their babies want to come out this way. Most babies sit in the womb in this position, but two thirds spontaneously flip head down before they are to be born – this probably has more to do with finding more room for their bodies as the grow larger. Experts say that your partner should begin doing a simple little exercise in the eight month of pregnancy that will help turn the baby. She is supposed to put pillows under her hips and lie flat on her back on the floor. The success rate of making the position change is an outstanding 89%.

Born in the Caul

When a baby is born in the amniotic sac it is called being born in the caul. The membranes balloon out of the vagina as the baby is born, enveloping the baby's face and body as birth occurs. There is no danger of the baby drowning as long as the umbilical cord is pulsing, the baby is getting oxygen. Care providers generally go ahead and tear the membranes when they appear, so as not to be splashed upon with a sudden rupture. A baby born in the caul is known as a caulbearer. Being born in the caul is seen as a positive and an omen of good fortune in most cultures. During the medieval time period an association was found between babies born in the caul and long term survivability. If your child was born in the caul, it rarely perished. There may be good reason for this connection. Remember that the baby is completely sterile until it is born and then within minutes it is covered with microbes. A baby born in the caul remains in sterile conditions through the birth canal and birth escaping being exposed to bacteria in the vagina.

Steady Evaluation

In the Birth Machine all complications are considered pathological. This is especially true about the length and time of labor. Some complications are nothing more than normal variations, which occur in the way birth happens. Once a complication occurs, and you are in the birth machine, you will soon see that interventions are the standard. In the medical model, birth is always a potential emergency. You should know that after your partner has reached 4 to 5 centimeters dilated, that the slowest progress of labor is over.

<u>Time of Birth</u>

Babies are born at all sorts of times prior and after due dates. Only a small percentage of women deliver at this time when we use that estimate of 280 to 288 days. Some women birth all their children late or early, and it may be a mixed bag. Complications with birth generally are suspect when labor begins three weeks early or two weeks late. Before you consent to induction at the later dates, make sure all the factors for ripeness of the cervix, etc. have been taken care of. The Bishops scale delineates the fact that the conditions have to be right or inductions fail. Also remember, once interventions start, they are apt to be followed by other interventions. That is how birth is handled in the birth machine. If on the other hand you are out of the hospital, your care provider will generally work on alternative approaches to interventions.

<u>Anemia</u>

Anemia is the reduction of hemoglobin found in our blood. Hemoglobin is an iron containing protein that carries oxygen throughout the body. When a woman is anemic her cells have difficulty dispersing oxygen throughout the body and to the brain. When a woman is pregnant this challenge becomes even more pronounced because the developing fetus is dependent upon receiving its oxygen from the mother's blood stream exchanged through the placenta. Anemia compromises her ability to oxygenate the baby and places her at greater risk to hemorrhage after a birth.

Some symptoms of anemia are fatigue, weakness, headache, reduced work capability and a decreased ability to maintain body temperature. The placenta sizes of mothers who are anemic are smaller in size than mothers who are not. Anemia is diagnosed when hemoglobin concentration is less than 11 grams per 100 ml of blood. When anemia is detected it must be turned around as soon as possible. The fact that a woman is anemic places her in a high risk pregnancy category because of the effect that anemia has on the function of the placenta. Women who are anemic are more likely to have a premature birth or low birth weight baby.

The most common cause of anemia is known as iron deficiency anemia. With careful and thorough consideration of a diet and supplementing with iron supplements this form of anemia can often be turned around. Foods rich in iron are clams, iron fortified breakfast cereals, tofu, lentils, eggs, chicken, legumes and dried fruit (Swinney 2000). Iron can be absorbed more readily when it is consumed with vitamin C. For example you can couple orange juice with a course of meat, or eating meat with spaghetti sauce. Some iron can also be captured by cooking and preparing food in iron cookware. For example spaghetti sauce cooked in a glass pan contains about 3mg of iron. The same spaghetti sauce prepared in an iron skillet may contain nearly 80mg of iron. Iron supplements come in differing forms a pleasant means of supplementing iron is by taking a liquid herbal form of iron. So many midwives have achieved good results with such a liquid herbal preparation that it earned the title of "corpse reviver." The more quickly that anemia can be turned around the more quickly the woman will be feeling better.

Placenta Delivery

After the baby is delivered, the placenta has to be delivered, and there can be problems that arise like part of the placenta does not deliver. These are times that medical care is necessary. You may find that unless there is heavy bleeding, usually the placenta will deliver easily. In a condition called Placenta accrete. The placenta becomes deeply implanted in the uterus, and usually requires a hysterectomy, but the condition has been very rare. Midwifery Today reports, the following:

> Statistics indicate that placenta accreta was a rare occurrence from 1930 to 1950—approximately one case in more than 30,000 deliveries. From 1950 to 1960 the number increased to one in 19,000 and by 1980 to one in 7,000. The most recent information suggests that the incidence has now risen to one in 2,500 deliveries.

Chapter 17: The Ways of Natural Childbirth

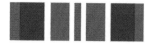

Natural childbirth advocates believe firmly in the physiological design of birth. This fundamental belief in the design of woman is championed ardently and passionately by its proponents. The holistic philosophy as mentioned before stresses this idea. Therefore, when natural childbirth is discussed, the process of birth is described in terms of the function and design of a woman's reproductive and birthing physiology. True natural childbirth means having a vaginal birth without any interventions like IVs, pit, forceps, vacuum extraction, amniotomy, or drugs.

Birth is Labor Intensive

If possible, labor is central in birth. The sensations of stretching and joints adjusting and the baby's head twisting through the birth canal is all related to this – causing discomfort, strain and pain. We men have little to compare with. About the only thing we can look at is lifting weights or performing a marathon. What makes it so different is that the conscious mind is not in control of the muscles doing all the hard work; this dilemma causes mental anguish as well.

In natural childbirth the fact is that progress is felt. The adjustments and the positions are all about feeling. What is incredible is that in birth just as a women has to be brought to orgasm in sexuality, she must be given the same security and privacy of sexuality to be able to open up to the birth process. As matter of fact in some aborigine cultures orgasm is not considered the end of the sexual experience the birth of a child is considered the culmination of the sexual union.

Both men and women release a surge of oxytocin naturally to be able to have an orgasm. In birth the same thing holds true. The woman's body has to in a way ejaculate the baby (fetal ejection reflex). For a very small amount of women, the same physiological sensations of orgasm occur when birthing. The point here is that birth is a sexual expression, and some women cannot birth until they feel safe and open, meaning intrusions and interferences can impede the natural course of labor, especially near the end when the baby is pushed out.

Your partner needs to be protected while she is birthing, she will not be talking much when the labor is in the intensity stage. Don't be asking her, or let anyone ask her, questions during this time period. That is when you know the baby is really coming. You know that when she is so absorbed in her birth work that she zones out. You (or another party) need to let her not be interrupted – stop intrusions, especially unwanted visitors or turning on the TV. She has to be able to focus through each contraction. Generally, there are hours and hours of first stage labor. This time is disconcerting for most women. Just think that you are there for the long run.

Early on, don't pay too much attention. Early labor takes a while. Only pay attention when things get intensified. Walk with her. Hold her. Comfort her. Think of this as an exciting time together. Treat her lovingly and tenderly.

Now, we aren't ever going to understand the feelings of birth, but apparently when a woman resists the contractions, she is not letting herself birth. Accepting the contractions and riding them out as if they are waves has been reported as the ideal way of managing the second stage. The intensity builds in natural labor as opposed to the magnified intrusion of induction agents like pitocin. As the intensity builds, you can gage the coming of the birth.

Nothing should be done quickly. Everything should be done to pace the birth. That's why you avoid the interventions. They speed things up and out of control. Even the baby does better if things aren't abrupt. Nothing is worse for a birth that your partner becoming tensed up or scared. Your partner needs to let the uterus have its way. Once she lets it take over, when she trusts its natural design, she can relax more with each contraction, so that even the strain diminishes.

Henci Goers, in her book Obstetric Myths Versus Research Realities, writes the following about how pain is part of the birth process:

> In fact, the pain and stress of non-medical labor have value. The stress hormones produced in response to labor, adrenaline and noradrenaline, trigger the final preparation of the fetal lungs to breathe air, mobilize fuel for energy, and, by shunting fetal blood away from the extremities and to the brain and heart (exactly opposite of the effect in adults), protect the fetus against hypoxia (oxygen lack) during labor (Lagercrantz and Slotkin 1986).

> Nerves in the cervix, and later the pelvic floor muscles and vagina, transmit stretching sensations as well as pain. These stretch receptors signal the pituitary to produce more oxytocin, which increases the tempo of the labor, causing further cervical dilation. Once the cervix is completely open and the head distends the pelvic floor and vagina, surges of oxytocin are produced, creating the urge to push. Numb the nerves with an epidural, and you also wipe out the positive feedback

mechanism (Johnson and Everitt 1988; Bates et al. 1985; Goodfellow et al. 1983).

Pain guides the mother. Commonly, the positions and activities she chooses for comfort are also those that promote good labor progress or help shift the baby into the right position for birth. Remove the pain, and you kill that feedback mechanism too.

The pro-epiduralists see the mother as needing rescue, but in reality her body prepares her to meet labor's challenge. Stress hormones give her stamina. By the time of the birth, endorphins, the body's natural painkillers, are found at levels 30 times higher than in nonpregnant women, and levels can be 20 times higher in women with prolonged or difficult labors as in uncomplicated labors (Jimenez 1988). Endorphins, produced in response to pain and stress, are also mood elevators. They are responsible, for example, for "runner's high." Oxytocin has mood-elevating and amnesiac properties too (Fuchs 1990).

Unlike epidurals, natural childbirth strategies facilitate labor both physiologically and psychologically. They raise endorphin levels, whereas epidurals reduce them (Jimenez 1988). They give the mother knowledge, skills, and confidence. Studies show that the key to a positive labor experience is mastery-a sense of control over events. With an epidural, control is completely given over to medical staff (Simkin 1991; Humenick 1981; Humenick and Bugen 1981).

What is important from that passage is that the natural issues of birth show that the whole process is interconnected. It is that the woman's body is doing things in response to other things which makes natural birth possible. To interfere with the process is to tamper with the design.

Believing is Paramount

Since birth is such a powerful event and one that can only happen so often in you and your partner's life together, believing in her ability to birth natural is probably the most important part of your place in the scheme of things. You really don't have much to do with the rest. Just think of birth in terms of running that marathon. If you were half way through, and you felt like you couldn't do it, and someone said, "Hey, dude, you don't have to run this race. Why don't you just jump in the car and we'll drive you to the finish." How would you feel? Natural childbirth is just as intensive and requires fortitude. Telling your partner you don't believe she can do it is about the worst possible thing you can do.

You ability to encourage your partner, to help her learn to trust her body is primarily what we're speaking of. You have been reading about childbirth, looking at the way it is handled. You've seen what the medical model is about and you know that natural childbirth inside that model is anything but natural, so it is your choices that make the difference. If you don't believe, you can't be supportive. That is why identifying your philosophical position is and aligning your position to your partner's position is so very important. As a father, you need to learn how to make two minds into one, and your kids will test that concept perpetually. The more connected you are with your partner the stronger you are in the face of pressure. Birth is all about handling pressure.

Birthing without Drugs

Not every birth even at home can avoid the need for drugs. If you birth in the hospital, drugs can be a constant focus. Most doctors prescribe drugs to help alleviate our pains and troubles. So it is very difficult to avoid them unless you are giving birth away from the medical model, at home or an alternative birth center.

But, in the holistic model that promotes natural childbirth, drugs are not relied upon. Drugs are not natural and they affect babies and mothers adversely. That can actually make drugs an enemy, especially if it interferes with the processes of birth.

A friend would be water – as in pools to birth in. Another friend is the constant care of a Doula, labor assistant or midwife. Friends are social supports, providing love and encouragement. Friends help eliminate the stress and they sooth the soul. Friends do not damn or ridicule you if you don't do as they say either.

Woman who birth naturally, without interfering drugs, will find that their babies are livelier and healthier. Many of the babies in the hospital suffer from higher rates of strep B infection, especially if they come out drugged. These babies go through the birth canal flaccid and unable to move normally. Their eyes may not be able to close. The risk is getting bacteria in their eyes that can cause blindness. They may not be able to close their mouths either. These types of risks are reduced considerably when a baby is strong and healthy.

Midwives report that when they lay a newborn (undrugged) on its mother's abdomen that the baby can maneuver itself by creeping upward until it finds the breast to suckle.

Birth as a Long Run

After having been to several births, and seen the long hours that pass in this physically draining event, birth looks much more like an Ironman competition. There are stages. There are shifts in focus. A woman usually changes her diet and exercise patterns before birth. She must be coached and stimulated to take care of the developing child within. Birth statistics show that healthier women deliver healthier babies.

As previously touched upon, when women are not allowed to eat or drink during their labor, that this in itself brings further complications. To give birth naturally without interventions, a woman has to be getting nourishment and must keep hydrated. If she is walking around for hours and changing positions, she is going to get tired out eventually when deprived of food and water.

When we exercise, we drink energy drinks fortified with electrolytes, so should a woman in birth. She is laboring – remember labor means work!

Stages of Natural Labor and Delivery

Nesting Instinct

Nesting is a phenomenon that occurs a short time before delivery where a woman becomes obsessed about the cleanliness or order of her household. Genny explains it was just a couple of days before our fourth child was born when I had to get up at 4 in the morning to mop our kitchen floor. When you observe odd behavior regarding domestic duties that boarder on obsessive around forty weeks you can be encouraged that labor is eminent. This nesting urge is a primal instinct. Other women about to deliver have been known to scour their entire households with a tooth brush, and to insist on new bed linens and towels though there is nothing wrong with the linens on hand. The best thing for you to do is remain good humored and encouraged that the nesting urge is associated with the onset of labor. The mother bird simply needs her nest to be in tip top condition before her baby arrives.

First Stage Beginnings

Usually when your partner gets up near her due date or up to two weeks after, she is going to see some signs of the impending birth. Often the first sign is your partner losing her mucous plug, which covers the opening of the cervix during pregnancy. This is a sign that the cervix is softened up and readying for the birth.

Rupture of Membranes / Water Breaking

One of the first events of labor may be the breaking of the water or rupture of membranes. The amniotic sac that has surrounded the baby during the course of the pregnancy bursts. Water bags rupture first in about 10% of births. 95% of these go into labor within 24 hours. A higher percentage of women's membranes rupture while they are laboring. We suggest that if your partner is concerned about her water breaking in public in the last days of pregnancy that she carry around with her a large mason jar of pickles and should she be caught with her membranes rupturing in public she can quickly throw her jar of pickles down and the public will be none the wiser. –We are only kidding. We do not want anyone to lacerate their foot.

Contractions

This is the most common way for labor to begin. The muscles of the uterus are usually being prepared way in advance, and the cervix is being softened up. Contractions are the force that pushes the baby down and forward, and stretches and opens the lower uterine segment called the cervix. Think of the cervix as the door of the uterus.

Early Labor

½ minute long, 10 minutes or so rest between

This is generally the beginning of the effacement and dilation of the cervix up to about 3 centimeters. This can take forever. You and your partner need to ignore most of this time especially when it is taking a long time. False labor can seem like early labor, but it will eventual peter out. Being vertical helps strengthen the effect of the contractions. If it is during the middle of the night, have your partner go back to sleep. Some women get an adrenaline rush, so try to calm her down. The energy needs to be saved for the long run. If her belly isn't getting hard to the touch and the contractions aren't running about three minutes apart don't be concerned with the speed of the birth. Your partner's body is just adjusting the cervix, thinning it out and opening it a bit. In a one-hour period of time, your partner may have three minutes of contractions and 57 minutes of peace.

Middle or Active Labor

1 minute long, 2 ½ minutes or more rest between

This moves the cervix from 3 centimeters to 8. Generally this takes on average about 12 hours. For those progressing slowly, the good news is that as long as progress is happening, a long slow labor is not a problem. Remember the cervix has to become fully effaced and stretched out before the baby can come through the birth canal.

Progress is very variable in this part. Sometimes women dilate one centimeter per hour in a nice consistent pattern. Other times, the progress can jump 5 centimeters in one hour. Even if you get to 8 centimeters, you still have some time before the birth. The longer you wait to arrive at a hospital in labor to birth, the more interventions you avoid. Remember if you arrive at the hospital at less than 4 or 5 centimeters dilated you can always leave and return later on in labor.

Transition

The last couple centimeters of dilation occur as the contractions are reaching their peak in performance. The rests and the contractions are equal in length and your partner is at her most tired. At this point many women really don't want to ever go through childbirth again. They get shaky, nauseous, and irritable. This step takes the most coaching to help her stay focused and determined. It usually lasts only an hour, for once the cervix opens up the baby can begin to descend through the birth canal.

Second Stage Last Big Effort

The second stage is when your partner will have to push the baby out. Women usually know when they feel the urge to push. Sometimes the great push takes only several minutes, but depending on your partner's state of mind and body after the first stage, she may be pretty tired out. Many women feel like they will burst open during this. The intensity is immeasurable. There is a burning feeling and an involuntary urge to expulse the baby.

The emergence of your child usually starts with a head of hair pushing through, all covered in shiny amniotic fluids. That is the crowning. Then the head pops out and usually, in a very short time the torso slides right out. This is it. There is your baby. No words can really tell the story. Everyone beams about it. The emotions run very high. It's like a big wonderful sigh. The cord is cut; the baby takes its first breaths -- sometimes its mouth and nose first have to be cleared of mucous. For us guys we may stand there and think it is all over, but the third act follows.

Third Stage
Just as your partner had to grow a baby, her body had to create a new bodily organ to feed the baby, and the sack to carry the baby, etc. So once the baby is out, she can hold her baby and even breastfeed the baby.

Stimulating the nipples helps to produce oxytocin to help her body to release the placenta that is still attached inside her uterus.

Birth with a Midwife

Midwives generally go through the whole birth with a woman. They are there to sit through the labor. Usually they work in tandems, or they work with a birth assistant or apprentice midwife. These women will take turns sitting with your partner through the long night. They provide a knowledgeable person the whole time.

Their main goal is to support your partner emotionally, and to hold her and comfort her during the labor process. They wipe up the fluids that drip and give your partner back rubs and suggest to her when she should try something new. The point is that the anguish and trial of labor is to be gone through together.

Midwife means with woman. Women who take on a midwife take on a wholly different style of care. The women who work as midwives see a completely different type of childbirth than what is going on in the hospitals. The individual woman and her partner are much freer to express birth as they feel. They are able to touch, caress, and do what they want.

There is no time limit on when the baby has to be born as long as mother and baby are doing fine. Ideally, an holistic midwife will not introduce a procedure to speed up the labor. They let things go naturally without drugs, without pressure, without intervention. Midwives just sit through the birth. They check vital signs, blood pressure; they look at fetal heart rates, lengths of contractions. Their number one sign of how labor is going is the laboring woman. They don't use machines to tell them the position of the baby; they use their fingers, hands, and ears.

Midwives are more often a soothing voice, one of confidence and reassurance. They believe in birth because they've done this umpteen times. Instead of prohibiting women from doing what they feel, they trust the woman's senses and feelings. The midwife reads her birthing mother, but doesn't dictate.

When you see what a midwife does, you will see that she is there for insurance, for her experience. She never undermines the woman's belief that she can have her baby naturally. She doesn't intercede at all unless a real complication arises. Many women could have their babies without help. It is a bodily process after all.

Midwives talk about dealing with the goop of birth. They wipe up the mess. They towel off the sweaty brow. They clean off the mucus. They discard the after birth. They wash the bedding, the linens and clean up the woman. When you look back on a midwife-assisted birth, you often don't think of the objective things they did during the birth, but rather the nurturing. You think more of holding hands, rubbing a tired back, and encouraging words.

Chapter 18: After the Landing

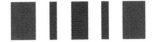

Looking For R&R?

No matter when the birth occurs, if you attended the birth you will be tired, but, remember you didn't run a race or climb any mountains, so you may have a few more yards to go before you take R&R. That baby is very vulnerable, and so is your partner. You need to think about whether everyone is settled and safe before you pull out your sleeping bag. Think of it as putting the planes in the hanger. You've landed, but your pilot just a bit longer.

At this point, you need to survey the landing site and check the participants. Depending on how smooth the landing and whether there was any damage, this process can be a short, easy time or a stressful one. The variables are many, but you can figure it out.

If the birth was traumatic, then you may find yourself both physically and emotional drained. Some men actually experience depression after such births. If your partner had a surgical procedure, and if some narcotics were involved, then you may be the only one alert enough to make good decisions. Just realize that though the birth is over, it isn't quite over. Once you have secured the perimeter, you can take a restful sleep, eat and unwind. This is your first day in this new state of life. You are now headed into possible new territory again, but the big landing is over, and you are still in one piece.

Calling in the Backups

After the birth has taken place, make a call to the leader of your backups. They will all want to share your joy and see the new arrival. Give everyone who went through the birth experience time to recuperate first. However, if you have to deal with something unexpected where either mother or baby needed a medic, then activate the part of your plan that calls in the backup team. If your care provider agreed to call in the troops, they relax and maintain your place as wingman. However, after a long difficult birth and then an unexpected result, you may be wiped out, so let others fill in. Backup are needed for at least a week even for a normal birth experience for at least a week while mother, baby and you adjust to your new living circumstances. However, if there is a prolonged recovery period like from a emergency surgery, then your backups may be needed for a longer time period. The harder the landing the more you will need to have your health care provider to bring in these helpers.

American health care usually does not provide overnight rooms for parents of babies who have serious complications. Not having adequate sleep after a birth is a disaster itself. We suggest having a hotel room nearby. Let others take care of you and step in to assist you and your family at this time, you will need it! If you don't go through the recovery, you will not be of much good no matter what transpires.

Debriefing

Just like astronauts, you will find the captain and the baby may have some more tests to run to ensure everything is going well. This shouldn't surprise you, but make sure you have a say in if the baby is going to be separated from you and your partner. Various concerns will be raised, and you 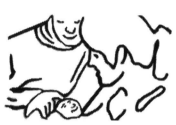 should have a basic knowledge of what you should be looking out for. Having basic understanding of newborn health issues is also in order.

Re Do

One cannot underestimate the poignancy surrounding the time of the birth and the time there after. You should work together to ensure that the environment surrounding these times is the one you both desire. These moments affect the quality of the marriage and family for a lifetime. This needs to be taken into consideration throughout the birth experience. It is not like going to a restaurant and having something go wrong with the service and simply musing to oneself that they can just do lunch over again.

An example of this situation occurred in our first birth experience. Genny had surgery and because of the anesthesia it was difficult for her to position our first child immediately after birth for breastfeeding. Our dear paternal friend was there to celebrate the joyous occasion of our birth. We were happy that he was there, but Genny needed to work on establishing the breastfeeding relationship with our first daughter (who by the way is named after this man we esteem so highly), and as much as we loved and respected this man, Genny could not find it in herself to ask him to leave at that time. Knowing and understanding what we do now about birth, we would be able to respectfully ask him to allow us the privacy necessary to establish breastfeeding. We didn't then however and we could never recapture those moments again where after the birth it is optimum to facilitate breastfeeding for the nourishment of the baby as well as for the involution of the uterus.

We certainly recognize that even with the best laid plans that there are many elements beyond our control. We would like to introduce and discuss the concept of the "re-do."

Frequently a family may have their hearts set on some detail of the birth experience whether it is the Mother touching the baby's head as it emerges, or of the Father and siblings cutting the cord. Perhaps it is bathing the baby for the first time yourself after the birth and something out of your control arises that presents an obstacle to that aspect of the birth that you had anticipated so fondly only to have your desires dashed by unseen circumstances. We wish to encourage you that though those exact moments may have been lost. You still may set aside some special time to create a "re-do" if you will, to create a special ceremony where you acknowledge the disappointment and take some action to bring healing to that area of loss.

If the disappointment was that you were not able to provide the first bath for your child, select an afternoon or time where you set about recreating that time with a special bath with your partner and health care provider if desired. Many alternative health care providers would be open to assisting you facilitate a recapturing of these lost moments, even some holistically minded physicians could understand such a need and be willing to work with you to provide for a healing from any element of disappointment arising from a birth experience. It is possible that a ceremony could be even more fulfilling than had the actual events gone off without a hitch. The important thing is that there be peace and resolve from disappointing events in order to pave the way for establishing optimum relationships within your family for the years to come.

PKU Test

You can wait for a week or two for this test that detects a rare enzyme deficiency. Blood is taken from the heel. The test is not accurate until the baby is digesting proteins, so wait.

Circumcision

If it is in your faith, this should wait until eight days after birth. It is not necessary in anyway physically, but it may be a spiritual or religious decision.

Registering the Baby

If you birth in the hospital, these procedures are routine. If not, don't forget that that state requires all children born to have a birth certificate.

Vitamin K

A baby begins to produce vitamin K at around 8 days old. Vitamin K is a precursor to the clotting factors found in blood. In the United States as well as other industrialized nations it is customary for the newborn infant to receive a shot of Vitamin K after the birth. There is a bleeding disorder that can appear in the first week of life in a newborn called hemorrhagic disease of the newborn (HDNB), or Vitamin K deficiency bleeding (VKDB). This disorder is extremely rare and has been found to be easily prevented by the routine injection of Vitamin K at the birth. In the United States the routine administration of vitamin K after the birth has made the occurrence of VKDB rare. The prevalence of VKDB is reported from 0.25 -1.7% (St. John 2006). If the birth has been a particularly traumatic birth with instrumental delivery such as with forceps or vacuum extraction and facial bruising occurs, it is a good idea to receive this prophylactic dose of vitamin K. Also if the baby is sick or will need corrective surgery, the vitamin K injection speeds the body's production of vitamin K. We find it interesting the correlation between the body's beginning the production of vitamin K on day 8 and the Jewish Rite of circumcision under the Abrahamic Covenant found in the T'nach (Genesis 17:9-14) that dictates a male child should be circumcised on the 8th day of life.

The Umbilical Cord Stump

With in days after birth the umbilical cord stump will dry up and fall off. Until then the care of the stump is quite simple. All you need to do is keep it clean and dry. At each diaper changing you may swab the umbilical stump with a cotton ball saturated with alcohol. You will wipe around the stump and it's top. The alcohol will encourage the stump to dry off and will effectively keep the area around the stump clean.

Low Birth Weight

Underdeveloped newborns often have issues with respiration. Newborns are more susceptible to infection.

Other Newborn issues

- Failure to breathe properly is marked by the following:

(a) Blue Skin, (b) Grunting during exhalation, (c) Body is pale or limp, (d) Gasping for air, or (e) Retraction of chest

- Jaundice (yellowed skin color) in the first 24 hours after birth or through the first week
- Lack of responses such as nursing
- Heartbeat lower the 100 beats per minute
- Convulsions
- Vomit that has bile in it
- Bloody defecation
- Obvious birth defects

Going Home

Sometimes you think you'll never get home – if you aren't there already. You will have car seat to install and for first timers that can be a challenge. Fire services, police services and state troopers often can provide help for those who are ignorant of how one of these contraptions works. Don't sweat it, but ducktaping the kids to the backseat doesn't work. Also you'll need a back seat so use a taxi if you drove the MG.

The First Weeks

You may have a great sense of pride and joy with this new little package in your life. You may want to sit and cuddle with the baby, but remember you are the wingman. Follow the captain's lead by providing that she gets just as many hugs and kisses. It's a pattern you set, so make sure you take care of number one, her. The more you love up on her the better for the child. Just spread the love.

Again depending on the type of landing you have just gone through, you will find that you are needed in many new ways. If you have an extended stay in the hospital, then you have that to deal with. If you stayed at home, then totally different circumstances, but one thing is for sure, that newborn is going to change the way you and your partner live, especially in how you sleep.

We have four children, and each one had a distinct personality, which manifested itself in how they slept. One child almost never slept solidly through a night until after age five. This child has today a high-strung psyche. He requires a great deal of tender care. His brother is and was just the opposite. He requires little attention, slept through the night after the first week, and actually gives more attention to others.

You will not be able to sleep or eat or anything as you did before. The child is going to demand attention and take a great deal of focus from the relationship with your partner. You should realize now that your partner can never be looked at the same way. There is now a child attached to her side. She is now a mother, and you are also not the same, you are a dad. You each have been promoted and with promotion comes greater responsibility.

New Team Member

Everyone grew up with a different family. Some of us never had any siblings. Some of us had sixteen. So when you have a baby, you are a family. A couple's relationship changes when this new team member arrives. Any change will mean that you will have to change.

Look at playing basketball. You can be the killer player, play great D and score from downtown. You might even dunk. But just keep adding players and see how that affects things. That star player who no one can guard gets his come-uppance when sunk in the mesh of a zone, or when he never gets the ball. Team sports are usually something we are familiar with. But adding a child into your relationship has both positives and negatives.

Back to Flying

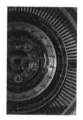

Your sexual appetites may have been stymied during the pregnancy, and birth sometimes totally takes you out of physical contact for some time. Your engines may still run at the same rpms, but you may have to avoid contact yourself, especially if your partner has some stitches or a surgical wound to heal. Then, you have the fatigue and the change of having to care for a child.

It is worst for you if you get aroused then for your partner. You are like the microwave. Your stimulation takes seconds – like boiling water. She is more like starting up the barbeque. Give it some time. Watch and wait. These changes are hard on her too, so you need to give her room to recuperate from the birth.

Physically, depending on the birth, your partner's sexual drive may not bounce back as a variety of emotional variables come to play. You will find that you must just relax. She may be giving so much energy in nurturing and caring for the baby, that she is touched out. She needs space. She may not be able to handle any sensual activity, being tired and worn down. The more you do to lighten the load for your partner and the more tenderness you show her the better the odds for flights to resume. For men sexuality is more spontaneous, but for women it is more of the nurturing and emotional expression. Try holding the baby often giving her the opportunity to take a bath or do some other relaxing activity.

Our recommendations for improving the intimacy at home: cuddle, hug and kiss, but stay affectionate and not erotic. Let her tell you at her pace when that should shift. Help out with the baby, and that means changing diapers, doing baths. Your partner, if nursing, will spend a load of time with this child. She will often get touched out. It is like her whole attention will be absorbed with the baby, and she will need serious breaks. That may mean you take the child, and she takes some time out. Take as much of the load as possible. This will help her recuperate. It takes a great deal of energy to feed the child and attend to its needs. Do everything you can. Showing her your support and shoring her up at this time where the demands of the newborn are so many will be more valuable to her and to the longevity of your family than you can ever imagine.

Once the Schedule is Made

The chaos of meeting the baby's demands will tire both of you out. Many nights of interrupted sleep are common. The baby will cause you and your partner to jockey schedules. You may even have to alter your own work schedule to allow for the care of the child – many employers offer paternity leave these days. But once there is some consistency, make your partner feel like a loved and cherished woman. Do something for her as often as you can think of it. Stop by a florist or the grocery and grab a bunch of fresh flowers. Buy a pretty gown. Get her a piece of jewelry. Tell her by actions that you love her.

Many times, due to the bustle of having a newborn, we spend most of our attention on the child's needs. But, the mother is the support system for the baby and ensuring she doesn't get overwhelmed or depressed should be your chief concern. You are designed to love the woman, and she may really need the support when she is burning the midnight oil caring for a child. This becomes magnified when a baby gets sick.

So be at your best. This is where you really make the difference. You really had little to do with her uterus doing its job. But, as the wingman, you just persist a little longer, and everything settles down. It's like you spent a quarter of the fuel to land this baby, so you should stay airborne until you are sure, absolutely that everything has been secured.

After Surgery

There are a few things you should be aware of if your partner had a cesarean. Many people forget that a cesarean section is not only a birth, but is also major abdominal surgery. Remember we covered post partum depression being rooted in expectations. So if your partner did not get the birth experience she signed up for, you know she is going to be wiped out. Her body and her mind are going to need some serious healing. She won't be able to pick up anything heavy due to the staples and stitches. She is also not going to be able to handle any emotionally draining activities. The recovery from surgery should be carefully observed. Infections can occur, so help your partner to deal with all that comes up, besides the weight of handling the strain of the baby. Think of an emergency surgery in these terms: If birth is a marathon race, what would it be like if you had an emergency knee repair at the 24th mile post. How would this affect you?

If you have had a major surgery, you will know that morphine is a narcotic that can make you feel no pain, but as soon as it wears of, you feel like you can't survive without pain relief. A few years ago, Phil split his cartilage in his knee and had surgery. At first he walked around and didn't need those crutches. The minute the morphine wore off, wham. It was like someone had hit him in the knee with a baseball bat.

You need to be in alignment with her feeling. If she is upset, comfort her and be understanding. Confirm her feelings. This is the best way of being supportive emotionally.

So if your partner had surgery, more will be expected of you at home. You will have to provide a great deal of emotional and physical support. You may have to cook all the meals and do all the laundry and anything else that comes up beyond just having to adjust to a new little baby's crying voice in the night.

Learning the New Instruments

As mentioned, the child begins seeking its own pattern and schedule, and that this is a function of its personality and level of health. So since the child cannot talk and barely can communicate, you will soon learn that it will be like a new set of instruments that you have to learn.

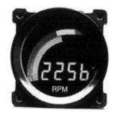

Crying is a variable. There are many cries and it's really hard to make them out at once. There are cries of distress and cries of wet or hungry.

The baby doesn't like pain, so it will let you know when life isn't quite comfortable. Some people think that you need to control the baby and ignore those cries. That is known as detachment parenting style. You control the feedings and the holdings, etc. Then there is a style in which you let the baby's needs control the arrangement. When the baby yells out for support, you find what it needs and take care of it. It takes some discernment to learn what these cries mean, but the baby has little else to offer. It requires your intelligence to pick out the differences as subtle as they first appear.

What is great about finding a clue to these obtuse signs is they will help you also discern when things aren't right. Babies are vulnerable to colic and sickness. Realizing a change in things helps you know when something out of the ordinary is happening. Having a pediatrician around to ask questions to will be of great benefit. A baby will cry, and your taking care of its needs will bring peace and harmony. Once you have exhausted rocking, feeding, changing, holding and warming – covering the physical needs – you will find that that is when you need expert advice.

If you choose to detach, then, you may be sending the message to your child that their needs are not important. But that is up to you and your personality and your choice of parenting style. No one can tell you how to handle these things, but babies cry, and that is how they communicate need. They also communicate contentment and happiness later on as the gurgle and smile and laugh.

One of the chief wonders of bringing a child into the world is watching those developmental milestones. They are a joy. They will continue to remain a joy as your child grows and is able to communicate to you they love you throughout y life. As long as you are meeting your child's needs, you will see love reciprocated. We suppose this is a very fundamental part of all of life. Give unselfishly and unconditional, and you will be given to.

Appendix A: Interviewing a Physician

Before you commit to a service provider, you need to learn if they fit your needs. Ask the questions below of potential physicians, and you will learn whether or not they fit you and your partner's needs.

Education and Philosophy

Where did you train? How long have you been in practice? Who are your partners in the practice? Will other doctors be involved in my partner's prenatal care or possible at out birth? How many births have you attended? Are you board-certified in obstetrics or family practice?

What is your philosophy about birth?

Expenses

What are your fees? What are the facility fees for the hospital? Are there any possible extra costs — for example for tests or anesthesia services — that I should know about?

Do you accept my insurance? (Name your insurance provider)? Check with your insurer to confirm this physician and his associates are covered!

If my insurance does not cover your services, are there alternative means of payment like time payments?

Prenatal Care and Childbirth Education

Does you office recommend childbirth education classes? Who do you recommend? Do you have a preferred style of childbirth you feel comfortable with? (Like Lamaze)

What schedule of prenatal visits do you recommend? What are the goals for prenatal appointments?

How would we know if our pregnancy becomes defined as "high-risk"? What things should we look out for?

Birth Participation Questions

Can I attend the birth? Can my partner and I bring friends and relatives to the birth? Is there any childcare available at the hospital? Can we bring our children to see the birth? Is there an age restriction? Can we videotape the birth?

We are considering using a birth attendant or a Doula, what are your recommendations?

We have read that there are many benefits to having a Doula.

Check-in

When do you recommend we come to the hospital to check in? How long is the check-in process? How much paperwork is there? Can we do some of the paperwork ahead of time?

What will hospital staff do once we are there? Are there any procedures?

How will you monitor the progress of our labor?

Who is going to monitor the baby during our labor? Do you prefer the Doppler, fetoscope or the EFM?

Doctor Policies

Do you order an IV while we are in labor or do you recommend liquid intake?

We have read that IVs are not appropriate as a routine practice because it limits the ability to move around in labor.

What do you think about eating during labor?

What positions do you recommend for birth?

Are there any limits the hospital puts on your ability to perform? Does the hospital have adequate trained staff to assist you in any way? Are there any better options you recommend or which make you more comfortable?

What is your policy if our water breaks before we get to the hospital? Are there any time limits? Or do you monitor for infection rather than use drugs to induce?

What is the percentage of surgical procedures you have done in the last 12 months? How many episiotomies have you done? How many c-sections? What is your VBAC rate? What about vacuum extractions or the use of forceps?

Dealing with Pain

What do you recommend we do to prepare for the stress and pain of labor?

Are there birthing tubs in the hospital? Can we walk around? Can my partner take a shower while she is laboring to reduce the pain? Can we have a chiropractic adjustment or a massage while in labor? Do you know of any other drug-free-pain relievers we could use?

What would happen if my partner decides to have an epidural?

Are other pain medications an option, and how do the affect the baby?

Do epidurals affect the baby?

Although opioids (narcotics) are available in many U.S. hospitals, the best available research suggests that they are not very effective in relieving pain and have risks for mothers and babies. Although nitrous oxide is not widely available in the U.S., the best available research suggests that it can provide helpful pain relief, with fewer unintended effects than either epidurals or opioids.

Care During Labor and Birth — Complications and/or Transfer

What percentage of your patients has a cesarean section?

Nearly one-fourth of birthing women in the U.S. have cesareans. This rate has steadily risen in recent years, and federal health objectives call for a reduction. A caregiver's style of practice can lead to a cesarean rate that is much higher or much lower than average.

If birth setting is not a "Level 3" (most specialized) hospital: What hospital would my baby be taken to, in the case of an unforeseen complication? What is the procedure for transfer?

Postpartum and Newborn care

What is your approach to newborn care? What are the routine procedures if a baby is healthy?

Does the birth setting where you practice place any limits on the care you would like to give in the newborn period? How do your views about newborn care match with the routines and policies of the setting where you practice?

How could we work together to ensure that breastfeeding gets off to a good start? Do you have special expertise in this area or work in collaboration with lactation consultants?

Breastfeeding offers important benefits. Breastfeeding support from informed and experienced individuals can help mothers establish and maintain breastfeeding.

Referrals

May I please have the names of some women who have recently received maternity care from you, for reference purposes?

Appendix B: Finding a Maternity Caregiver

Each area of North America developed slightly different resources available for pregnant women. Childbirth options in some places were very restricted historically. Now we are left with the situation as it currently sits. So where do you find information? Since most of us have access to the world wide web, you could use a plethora of resources available there. There are more materials out there than you want to read.

Many ways exist to find and get information about maternity caregivers in your area, including the following:

Contact your insurance company for a listing of service providers they cover: contact member services or customer service.

Do some research on the internet. One site that is very useful is www.childbirthconnection.org – on the left-hand navigation sidebar you will find "Choosing a Caregiver."

Ask new mothers in your area. Ask them about their experiences – see if they reveal their philosophy of birth and their care providers.

Obtain information and recommendations from area childbirth educators, Doulas, breastfeeding counselors, maternity nurses, and others who are familiar with maternity caregivers and women who have worked with them.

Finding a Nurse Midwife

At the website of the American College of Nurse-Midwives, you will find over 2,000 choices, broken down by state. The wed address is as follows:

http://www.midwife.org/find.cfm

Finding a Midwife

Certified midwives and direct entry midwives exist across the U.S. Funding one in your local area may require a little digging. As midwives are illegal in certain states, you have to use word of mouth often. However there are national resources to assist you. One is Citizens for Midwifery. This organization tracks where midwives are and what their legal status is. They also have a locator on the internet at the following address:

http://cfmidwifery.org/find

You can search a midwife locator on the Midwifery Today website at www.midwiferytoday.com. The link is located on the left-hand navigation bar on their web page.

The www.midwifeinfo.com site also has a midwife locator at the following internet address:

http://www.midwifeino.com/practitioners/

What is nice about their site is that it lists location and certifications of the practitioners listed.

You can get referrals to members of the Midwives Alliance of North America by calling toll-free: 888-923-MANA (888 923-6262) or sending an e-mail to info@mana.org.

Finding a Physician

The website of the American College of Obstetricians and Gynecologists is listed as www.acog.org and has a comprehensive directory of member obstetrician- gynecologists; (see "Find a Physician" on the home page -- http://www.acog.org/member-lookup/disclaimer.cfm). Visitors can search by town, zip code, or provider name. All members are board-certified and have active licenses to practice. The American Medical Association also has a web page located at http://www.ama-assn.org/.

Family Physicians are another source for doctors. The American Academy of Family Physicians website is located at http://www.aafp.org/online/en/home.html. For their locator:

http://familydoctor.org/online/famdocen/home/pat-advocacy/healthcare/836.html.

This site also lists useful information about pregnancy and childbirth at the following link:

http://familydoctor.org/online/famdocen/home/women/pregnancy.html.

Another group of physicians that deliver babies are osteopaths, also known as DOs. You can search a directory of osteopathic physicians on the website of the American Osteopathic Association. The directory includes information about practice specialty and educational background. Go to the following link for more information:

http://www.osteopathic.org/index.cfm?PageID=findado_main

Finding a Birth Center

Harder to find than a Doctor, Midwife or Doula will be finding a birth center. There are only about 200 in the United States. The American Association of Birth Centers provides a locator for all of the active centers at this address:

http://www.birthcenters.org/find-a-birth-center/

Finding a Doula

Several sites will direct you to finding a Doula in your area. The magazine Midwifery Today provides a locator at the following address:

http://www.findaDoulatoday.com/birthmarket/

Doulas of North America have a web site that lists a locator as well. 6400 Doulas are members of this organization. The locator is on their main web page on the left-side and is easily found: http://www.dona.org

Different Types of Caregivers

Professionals approach birth differently depending on their training and experience. OB/GYNs, family physicians and DOs are all doctors but have different philosophies about childbirth. Midwives also receive training that is at different points in the spectrum. Doulas are also becoming popular for those trying to have a more satisfying birth in the hospital. To clarify these distinctions you might read sections from the following books or web sites:

Joyce Barrett and Teresa Pitman. *Pregnancy and Birth: The Best Evidence: Making Decisions that are Right for You and Your Baby*. (Toronto: Key Porter Books, 1999). [See chapter 1.]

Henci Goer. *The Thinking Woman's Guide to a Better Birth*. (New York: Perigee Books, 1999). [See chapter 12.]

Dr. William Sears and Martha Sears. *The Birth Book: Everything You Need to Know to Have a Safe and Satisfying Birth*. (New York: Little, Brown & Company, 1994). [See chapter 3.]

Or use the website for Child Birth Connection at the following address:

http://www.childbirthconnection.org

Appendix C: Rights of Women

Women have only had the right to vote for about one hundred years. Women are still often considered second-class citizens. Maternity care brings out many of the old prejudicial attitudes in society. Every woman should be respected especially during carrying and delivering a baby, but such consideration is neglected especially in the medial world that is still dominated by men. Fortunately, society attitudes have shifted, and there are many legal precedents that now support women's rights. These rights continue to expand year after year. All women need to have access to health care before, during and after pregnancy and childbirth; yet no socialized form of medicine or governmental aid that insures this in the United States.

We have excerpted the following materials from The Maternity Center Association web pages with their permission.

Current Legal Rights

1. Every woman and infant has the right to receive care that is consistent with current scientific evidence about benefits and risks.

2. Every woman has the right to choose her birth setting from the full range of safe options available in her community, on the basis of complete, objective information about benefits, risks and costs of these options.

3. Every woman has the right to communicate with caregivers and receive all care in privacy, which may involve excluding nonessential personnel. She also has the right to have all personal information treated according to standards of confidentiality.*

4. Every woman has the right to full and clear information about benefits, risks, and costs of the procedures, drugs, tests and treatments offered to her, and of all other reasonable options, including no intervention.*

5. Every woman has the right to accept or refuse procedures, drugs, tests and treatments, and to have her choices honored. She has the right to change her mind.*

6. Every woman has the right to be informed if her caregivers wish to enroll her or her infant in a research study. She should receive full information about all known and possible benefits and risks of participation, and she has the right to decide whether to participate, free from coercion and without negative consequences.*

7. Every woman has the right to unrestricted access to all available records about her pregnancy, her labor, and her infant; to obtain a full copy of these records. If she does not understand the details, she may ask to receive help in understanding them.

8. Every woman has the right to receive maternity care that is appropriate to her cultural and religious background, and to receive information in a language in which she can communicate.

9. The right to receive full advance information about risks and benefits of all reasonably available methods for relieving pain during labor and birth, including methods that do not require drugs. She has the right to choose which methods will be used and to change her mind at any time.

10. The right to freedom of movement during labor. This means no tubes, wires, or other apparatus. She also has the right to give birth in the position of her choice.

Rights Not Won in Court Yet

1. Practices that have been found to be safe and beneficial should be used when indicated. Harmful, ineffective, or unnecessary practices should be avoided. Unproven interventions should be used only in the context of research to evaluate their effects.

2. The right to choose a midwife or a physician as her maternity care provider. Both caregivers skilled in normal childbearing and caregivers skilled in complications are needed to ensure quality care for all.

3. Every woman has the right to receive all or most of her maternity care from a single caregiver or a small group of caregivers, with whom she can establish a relationship. Every woman has the right to leave her maternity caregiver and select another if she becomes dissatisfied with her care.

4. Every woman has the right to information about the professional identity and qualifications of those involved with her care, and to know when those involved are interns, apprentices or in training.

5. Every woman has the right to receive maternity care that identifies and addresses social and behavioral factors that affect her health and that of her baby. She should receive information to help her take the best care of herself and her baby and have access to social services and behavioral change programs that could contribute to their health.

6. She should receive this information about all interventions that are likely to be offered during labor and birth well before the onset of labor.

7. Every woman has the right to have family members and friends of her choice present during all aspects of her maternity care.

8. Every woman has the right to receive continuous social, emotional, and physical support during labor and birth from a caregiver who has been trained in labor support.

9. Every woman has the right to virtually uninterrupted contact with her newborn from the moment of birth, as long as she and her baby are healthy and do not need care that requires separation.

10. Every woman has the right to receive complete information about the benefits of breastfeeding well in advance of labor, to refuse supplemental bottles and other actions that interfere with breastfeeding, and to have access to skilled lactation support for as long as she chooses to breastfeed.

11. Every woman has the right to decide collaboratively with caregivers when she and her baby will leave the birth site for home, based on their condition and circumstances.

Sources

The following sources have helped guide the development of this statement of rights:

American Hospital Association. A Patient's Bill of Rights, revised edition approved by the AHA Board of Trustees on October 21, 1992.

Annas, G. J. A national bill of patients' rights. New England Journal of Medicine338, (10) 695-699, 1998.

Annas, G. J. The Rights of Patients, second edition. Carbondale, IL; Southern Illinois University Press, 1989.

Boston Women's Health Book Collective. Section on "Child-bearing" and chapter on "The politics of women's health and medical care." In: Our Bodies, Ourselves for the New Century, New York: Simon & Schuster, 1998, pp. 433-543, 680-722.

Coalition for Improving Maternity Services (CIMS). The Mother-Friendly Childbirth Initiative, 1996. Available on Internet at: http://www.motherfriendly.org

Enkin, M., M.J.N.C. Keirse, M. Renfrew, and J. Neilson. A Guide to Effective Care in Pregnancy and Childbirth,second edition. New York: Oxford University Press, 1995.

International Childbirth Education Association, Inc. The Pregnant Patient's Bill of Rights.Minneapolis: ICEA, 1975.

President's Advisory Commission on Consumer Protection and Quality in the Health Care Industry. Appendix A. Address on the web: http://www.hcqualitycommission.gov/final/append_a.html

United Nations. Universal Declaration of Human Rights. Published by the United Nations, 1948.

Appendix D: Discomforts of Pregnancy

Discomfort	Onset	Remedy	Danger sign
Backache	Middle of 2nd trimester	▪ Good posture. ▪ Supportive shoes ▪ Avoid standing for long periods of time. ▪ Exercise at least three times a week ▪ Apply heat using warm bath soaks, warm wet towels, a hot water bottle or heating pad ▪ Give a back massage ▪ Rest	Consider whether continued back ache is actually premature back labor. If in doubt contact you health care provider.
Constipation	2nd or 3rd trimester	▪ Give adequate fluid intake (64 ounces of liquids) ▪ Prunes ▪ Fruits and veggies ▪ Adequate sleep ▪ Food with fiber ▪ Exercise ▪ When needed laxatives	No bowel movement for at least 7 days. Blockage could be possible, if laxatives don't work, consult health care provider
Distortions in Taste & Smell	Many women experience a heightened sense of smell as the first sign that they are pregnant. Occurs throughout the whole of a pregnancy.	▪ Suck ice chips ▪ Avoid strong odors such as alcohol, cleaners, cigarettes smoke, and strong cooking smells ▪ Fresh cool air, especially while eating.	Severe prolonged vomiting and dehydration, abdominal cramping, and fever. Generally being unable to keep solid food down for 24 hours, weight loss, ketones in urine can be used as signs that the nausea or vomiting is severe enough to warrant some treatment
Dizziness Faint-Light Headiness	1st,2nd and 3rd trimester	▪ Change positions slowly ▪ Body bolster pillow ▪ Rest on the side with leg supported by pillow	
Diarrhea	Early pregnancy	▪ Eat more dairy products ▪ Ensure fluid intake is sufficient	Dehydrated to the point of needing medical intervention
Hemorrhoids	Any time	▪ Avoid sitting on the toilet for long periods of time or straining ▪ Cold witch hazel pads ▪ Ice pack ▪ Avoid hemorrhoid medicines containing local anesthetics ▪ Warm baths ▪ Kegel exercises ▪ "doughnut" cushion	This may accompany constipation.
Fatigue	Fatigue occurs during the first	▪ Mild exercise and good nutrition	Severe fatigue can be

Discomfort	Onset	Remedy	Danger sign
	trimester for no known reason	▪ Frequent rest periods during the day ▪ Extra sleep	connected to anemia. When combined with sudden drops of blood pressure and chest discomfort, can mimic heart disease. Fatigue can also be caused by an infection. Fatigue is also a classic sign of depression so mood can be involved.
Gassiness and Heartburn	Anytime	▪ No greasy, fried or spicy foods.. ▪ Avoid both coffee and cigarettes ▪ Provide more but smaller meals each day ▪ Stay hydrated ▪ Try carbonated water ▪ Try yogurt or ice cream, ▪ Avoid acidic foods, such as citrus, tomatoes, red peppers, and chocolate	Consult with your health care provider before taking any antacids
Headache	Common in the 1st trimester	▪ Apply a cool or warm compress to the forehead or the neck ▪ Warm shower/ bath ▪ Massage ▪ Because low blood sugar can trigger headaches she should eat smaller more ▪ frequent meals to avoid headaches. ▪ If combined with exhaustion than sleep.	If she has headaches in the 2nd and 3rd trimester it could be a sign of pre-eclampsia. If headache comes after falling or hitting head, there is a serious problem. If nasal congestion with pain and pressure under the eyes could be sinus infection needing antibiotics.
Heart Palpitations		▪ When you feel your heart pounding, let go of tension throughout your body. Start at your head and relax each part of your body until you reach your toes. ▪ Take slow, deep breaths. ▪ Limit activities that require a lot of energy and effort.	Contact your health care provider if you feel your heart pounding often or irregularly.
Insomnia	3rd trimester	▪ Avoid caffeinated drinks ▪ Warm baths ▪ Massage and relaxation techniques.	It can negatively affect childbirth if woman goes into labor fatigued.

Discomfort	Onset	Remedy	Danger sign
		- Exercise that create physical tiredness. - Some herbal teas and homeopathics. - Regular sleep cycle. - Take actions to"set the stage for sleep" i.e Dim Lights, Relaxing Baths	
Itching	2nd and 3rd trimester	- Avoid mineral oil based skin lotions and harsh bath and laundry soaps - Increase intake of foods rich in vitamins A, D, and linolenic acids - Oatmeal baths - Natural fiber clothing - Avoid extreme temperatures - Humidifier	When fever or jaundice is involved could indicate more serious problem, consult your health care provider
Leg Cramps	2nd and 3rd trimester	- Leg stretches - Exercise regularly, Leg elevation. - Diet including both calcium and phosphorous, juices fortified with calcium. - During cramping try stretching and walking - A warm bath - Avoidance of prolonged standing and sitting cross legged.	A blood clot, can occur in 1 in 2000 pregnancies. It is accompanied by persistent pain and redness. It should not be massaged. Another problem that can occur is Thrombophlebitis which is an inflammation of the deep veins of the leg that can lead to a blood clot.
Moodiness	This occurs most often during the 1st and 3rd trimesters.	- She needs to be around supportive, sensitive and uncritical people. - Keep all conversation friendly, call for backup emotional support/help when fired upon. - Avoid major renovations or moves during pregnancy.	If emotions do not return to center, and there are uncontrollable crying, panic attacks, significant depression and or expressions of worthlessness, then seek professional help.
Morning Sickness	Occurs from 4-22 weeks with the prime time between 8 and 12 weeks. However, nausea and vomiting can occur at any time during a pregnancy.	- Reassurance that nausea in pregnancy is normal - Frequent small meals with easily digestible carbohydrates, low in fats. - Avoid strong smells and heavy food like meats. - Carbonated drinks. - Acupressure bands - Acupuncture - Homeopathic remedies: - Fresh air - Crackers	Look for signs of dehydration, as nutrients aren't being absorbed. Or for weight loss, poor appetite, and electrolyte imbalance. When she can't hold down food and has weight loss, then see you care provider.

Discomfort	Onset	Remedy	Danger sign
Nasal Stuffiness allergies Nose bleeds	It frequently starts in the third month of pregnancy, but may start earlier, and can last until delivery or even a few weeks afterward	▪ For nasal stuffiness: ▪ avoid irritants like aerosols, smoke, or temperature changes. ▪ Use steam via a bowl of hot water or a humidifier ▪ Stay hydrated ▪ As a last resort, ask a health care professional which medications would be safe to try ▪ For Nose Bleeds: ▪ Keep head higher than heart. ▪ Put pressure on bleeding nostril for five to ten minutes.	If stuffiness is accompanied by fever or signs of infection see a doctor. If nose bleeds don't stop after consistent pressure is applied after ten minutes then contact a healthcare professional.
Night urination	Occurs typically in 3rd trimester	▪ Practice kegel exercises and limit fluids during evenings and nights	If she has fever or pain during urination, both are signs of urinary tract infection.
Numbness Tingling of Hands and Feet	25% of pregnant women experience these symptoms; starting in 2nd trimester	▪ Avoid typing and gripping activities ▪ Paraffin bath ▪ Swimming as exercise	If accompanied by swelling could be sign of pre-eclampsia
Shortness of Breath		▪ Hold her arms over your head. ▪ Head elevated on pillows at rest or sleep ▪ Slow deep breathing when relaxing ▪ When stair climbing go slowly	
Skin changes	Can appear in 2nd trimester but usually in 3rd with most women	▪ Avoidance of sun or have her wear sunscreen ▪ Nutritionally folate is supposed to help reduce the problem	Moles that change color, size and border may indicate problems.
Sore and bleeding gums	2nd or 3rd trimester month of pregnancy	▪ Get a soft bristle tooth brush ▪ Brush gently ▪ Floss ▪ Sensitive style toothpaste ▪ Check your diet for adequate amounts of Vitamin C, a vital nutrient for tissue healing ▪ Use mouthwash to remove the blood taste	Gingivitis is a gum, infection and can lead to periodontitis where the infection can develop in the bone and other tissues If there is chronic gum disease (gingivitis) this brings up risks in pregnancy.
Swelling	Usually 2nd and/or 3rd trimester	▪ Avoid constrictive clothing ▪ Elevate legs	Could involve hypertension. If her face swells then could be a sign of pre-eclampsia

Discomfort	Onset	Remedy	Danger sign
		periodically • Lie down on one side • Find maternity abdominal support or girdle, to help take the pressure off the pelvic veins. • Exercise, especially swimming	
Uterine Contractions (Braxton Hicks)	Uterine contractions start about the 6th week of pregnancy that are sporadic and painless until the late into pregnancy when they increase in frequency, duration, intensity, and regularity	• Drink herbal teas which are for relaxing • Rest is important • Urinate frequently • Avoid nipple stimulation • Reduce contact with infants	If contractions come more than four to six per hour and they develop a consistent rhythm before the 37th week of pregnancy they may be a prelude to preterm labor. Contact your health care provider
Varicose Veins	Usually become visible during 3rd trimester	• Leg elevation and exercise • Support hoses. • Proper seating not cramping legs or pressing them into something hard. • Less time on feet.	Usually is cosmetic in nature and not causing further complications

Appendix E: Infertility & Infant Death Resources

The following list provides information about organizations that support families that have suffered the loss of an infant. They provide books, brochures, catalogues, special baby books and birth certificates, birth/death announcements, newsletters, support groups, help lines, conferences, workshops, etc. Also listed are any web sites or email addresses for those organizations.

Miscarriage or Stillborn Child

Centering Corporation
7230 Maple Street
Omaha, Nebraska 68134
(800) 218-0101
www.centeringcorp.com

National SHARE Office
402 Jackson Street
St. Charles, Missouri 63301-2893
(636) 947-6164
(800) 821-6819
www.nationalshareoffice.com

The Compassionate Friends
National Office
P.O. Box 3696
Oak Brook, Illinois 60522-3696
(630) 990-0010
www.compassionatefriends.org

RTS Bereavement Services
1910 South Avenue
La Crosse, Wisconsin 54601
(608) 775-4747
(800) 362-9567, Ext. 54747
www.bereavement.org

Pregnancy and Infant Loss Center
3210 Ewing Drive
Manuel, Texas 77578
www.pregnancyandinfantloss.org

A Place To Remember
1885 University Avenue, Suite 110
Saint Paul, Minnesota 55104
(800) 631-0973

Wintergreen Press
3630 Eileen Street
Maple Plain, Minnesota 55359
Phone and Fax: (612) 476-1303
www.wintergreenpress.com

Bereavement Publishing, Inc.
8133 Telegraph Dr.
Colorado Springs, Colorado 80920
(888) 604-4673
www.breavementmag.com

Bereaved Parents of the USA
National Headquarters
P.O. Box 95
Park Forest, Illinois 60466-0095
(708) 748-7672
www.bereavedpartsusa.org

Loss in a Multiple Birth

Center for Loss In Multiple Birth (CLIMB)
P.O. Box 91377
Anchorage, Alaska 99509
(907) 222-5321
www.climb-support.org

Christian Based Support

M.E.N.D. Mommies Enduring Neonatal Death
Christian nonprofit corporation with newsletter and website.
P.O. Box 1007
Coppell, TX 75019
(972) 506-9000
www.mend.org

Hannah's Prayer
Christian infertility, pregnancy loss, and early infant death support.
Quarterly newsletter (both e-mail and postal mail editions), and local
care/support group chapters.
PO Box 15053
Long Beach, California 90815
www.hannahsprayer.org

Caleb Ministries
Christian help for women dealing with infertility, miscarriage, stillbirth,
and early infant death (up through 1 year).
PO Box 470093
Charlotte, North Carolina 28247
(704) 841-1320
www.calebministries.org

High Risk Pregnancy

Sidelines National Support Network
(Supporting Women in High Risk Pregnancies)
P.O. Box 1808
Laguna Beach, California 92652
(888) 447-4754
www.sidelines.org

Elective Abortions (Fetal Anomalies)

Heartbreaking Choices
A book and website for parents who have interrupted their pregnancies
after prenatal diagnosis revealed severe fetal anomalies.
www.ourheartbreakingchoices.com

Sudden Infant Death Syndrome

National SIDS Foundation
1314 Bedford Ave., Suite 210

Baltimore, Maryland 21208
(800) 221-7437
www.firstcandle.org

Shaken Baby Syndrome (SBS)

National Center on Shaken Baby Syndrome
2955 Harrison Blvd. #104
Ogden , Utah 84403
www.dontshake.org

References

Articles and Books

Althabe, et al. *Caesarean section: The paradox*. The Lancet 2006. 368: 1472-3

American College of Obstetricians and Gynecologist, "Routine Ultrasound in Low Risk Pregnancy, ACOG Practice Patterns: Evidence –Based Guidelines for Clinical Issues, Obstetrics and Gynecology. August 1997

Anderson, G., et al. Early skin-to-skin contact for mothers and their healthy newborn infants. Cochrane Review Issue 1. Oxford England 2002

Anderson, Rondi. and Anderson, David. *The Cost Effectiveness of Home Birth Journal of Nurse-Midwifery*, Vol. 44, No. 1, January/February 1999.

Arms, Suzanne. Immaculate Deception II--A Fresh Look at Childbirth. Celestial Arts 1994 Berkeley, CA

Baldwin, Rahima, Special Delivery. Celestial Arts, 1990. Berkeley, CA

Banks, Amanda Carson. Birth chairs, midwives, and medicine. Jackson University Press. 1999. Jackson, MS.

Barrett, Joyce and Pitman, Teresa. Pregnancy and Birth: The Best Evidence: Making Decisions that are Right for You and Your Baby. Key Porter Books. 1999. Toronto

Bujold MD, Emmanuel, Gauthier MD, Robert J. *Should We Allow a Trial of Labor After a Previous Cesarean for Dystocia in the Second Stage of Labor?* Obstetrics & Gynecology 2001;98:652-655

Buckley Sarah, *Weighing the Risks: What You Should Know about Ultrasound.* Mothering Magazine 102 September – October 2000.

Caughey, et al. *Chorionic Villus Sampling Compared With Amniocentesis and the Difference in the Rate of Pregnancy Loss.* Journal of Obstetrics and Gynecology Vol. 108, No. 3 September 2006. 612-616

Caughey, et al. *Contemporary Diagnosis and Management of Preterm Premature Rupture of Membranes.* Reviews in Obstetrics & Gynecology. Vol 1 No. 1 2008 11-22

Cohen Nancy, Estner Lois, Silent Knife: Cesarean Prevention and Vaginal Birth after Cesarean. Greenwood Press. March 1983. Westport, CT.

Committee On Bible Translation, Holy Bible New International Version. Zondervan. 2001. Grand Rapids, MI

Davis-Floyd, Robbie E. Birth as an American Rite of Passage. University of California Press. 2004. Berkeley, CA.

Dick-Read, Grantly. Childbirth without fear; the principles and practice of natural childbirth. Heinemann. 1960. London.

Doss, et al. *The effect of the transition to parenthood on relationship quality: An eight- year prospective study.* Journal of Personality and Social Psychology. Vol 96(3), Mar 2009, 601-619

Eggerichs, Emerson, Love & Respect: The Love She Most Desires; The Respect He Desperately Needs. Thomas Nelson. September 2004. Nashville, TN.

Enkin, Murray, Keirse, Marc. J., Chalmers, Iain. A guide to effective care in pregnancy and childbirth. Oxford University Press. 1989. New York, NY.

Freeman Roger. Fetal Heart Rate Monitoring 3rd ed. Lippincott Williams & Wilkins 2003. Hagerstown, MD

Frye, Anne. Holistic Midwifery: A Comprehensive Textbook for Midwives in Homebirth Practice, Vol. 1: Care During Pregnancy. Labrys Press. 1998. Portland, OR.

Frye, Anne Understanding Lab Work in the Childbearing Year 4ed., Labrys Press. 1990. New Haven, CT.

Goer, Henci. *The Assault on Normal Birth: The OB Disinformation Campaign.* Midwifery Today. www.midwiferytoday.com/articles/disinformation.asp 2002

Goer, Henci. The Thinking Woman's Guide to a Better Birth. Perigee Books. 1999. New York, NY.

Goer, Henci. Obstetric Myths Versus Research Realities. Bergin & Garvey, 1995. New York, NY.

Gordis, Leon. Epidemiology. Saunders Publishers. 2004. Philadelphia. PA.

Gray John. Men Are From Mars, Women Are From Venus, Harper Collins 1992 New York, NY

Hales et al. *Influence of labor and route of delivery on the frequency of respiratory morbidity in term neonates.* International Journal of Gynecology and Obstetrics, 1993; vol. 43 pg 35-40

Hamilton et al. Births: Preliminary Data for 2007 National Vital Statistics Reports. U.S. Department of Health and Human Services Centers for Disease Control and Prevention National Vital Statistics System March 18, 2009

Harrison, Mitchell. A Woman in Residence. Random House. 1982. New York, NY.

Harvey, et al. *Suggested Limits to the Use of the Hot Tub and Sauna by Pregnant Women.* Canadian Medical Association Journal. 1981 July 1. 125: 50.

Haverkamp, et al. *The evaluation of continuous fetal heart rare monitoring in high-risk pregnancy.* American Journal Obstetrics and Gynecology. 1976; 125:310-320 (1)

Houser, Patrick. Fathers-To-Be Handbook. Creative Life Systems. 2009. South Portland, ME.

Hughey, Michael. Military Obsterics and Gynecology. Brookside Associates. 2005 Wilmette, IL

Jacobson, et al. *Opiate addiction in adult offspring through possible imprinting after obstetric treatment.* British Medical Journal. 1990 November 10. 301(6760): 1067–1070.

Johnson Robert, et al. Mayo Clinic Complete Book of Pregnancy and Baby's First Year William Morrow. 1994. New York, NY.

Kannan et al. *Maternal satisfaction and pain control in women electing natural childbirth.* Reg. Anesth. Pain Med 2001, 26: 468-72.

Kitzinger Shelia, The Complete Book of Pregnancy and Childbirth. Alfred A. Knopf. 1996. New York, NY.

Leboyer, Frederick. Birth without Violence. Knopf. 1975. New York, NY.

Lent Margaret. *The Medical and Legal Risks of the Electronic Fetal Monitor.* Stanford Law Review, Vol. 51, No. 4 (April 1999), pgs 807-837.

Maestas, Linda M. *The Effect of Prenatal Education on the Beliefs and Perceptions of Childbearing Women.* International Journal of Childbirth Education, Mar 2003, Vol. 18 Issue 1, pgs.17-21.

Menacker Fay. *Trends in Cesarean Rates for First Births and Repeat Cesarean Rates for Low-Risk Women: United States, 1990-2003.* National Vital Statistics Reports US Department of Health and Human Services. Vol 54, Number 4. September 22, 2005

Middleton Jane, Rapitis, George. The Healthy Pregnancy Cookbook: eating twice as well for a healthy baby. Hungry Minds. 2002. New York, NY.

Mishell Jr., Daniel, Management of Common Problems in Obstetrics and Gynecology 4th ed. Blackwell Publishing. April 2002. Boston, MA.

Newnham, J. P., et al., *Doppler Flow Velocity Wave Form Analysis in High Risk Pregnancies: A Randomized Controlled Trial.* British Journal of Obstetrics. 98, No. 10. 1991. 956-963.

Oxorn, Harry. Oxorn-Foote Human labor & birth. Appleton-Century-Crofts. Norwalk, Conn. 1986

Peterson Gayle & Mehl-Madrona Lewis. <u>Birthing Normally A Personal Growth Approach to Childbirth 2nd ed.</u> Shadow & Light December 1991 pg.11

Rooks Judith. <u>Midwifery and Childbirth in America.</u> Temple University Press. February, 1999. Philadelphia, PA

Rosegg, Susan M. <u>Natural Childbirth the Bradley Way</u>. Plume. 1996. New York, NY.

Ross, Michael. *Meconium Aspiration Syndrome—More than Intrapartum Meconium.* New England Journal of Medicine. September 1, 2005. No.9 volume 353:946-948.

Rothman, Barbara Katz, <u>In labor: Women and Power in the Birthplace.</u> W.W. Norton and Co. 1982. New York, NY.

Ryan Kenneth. *Giving Birth in America, 1988.* Family Planning Perspectives, Vol. 20, No. 6. Nov. - Dec., 1988, pp. 298-301

Schenker, et al. *Fetal Alcohol Syndrome: Current Status of Pathogenesis.* Alcoholism: Clinical and Experimental Research, 14 September/October 1990: 635

Scott, J., et al. Danforth's Obstetrics and Gynecology, 9th ed. Lippincott Williams and Wilkins. 2003. Philadelphia, PA

Sears, William and Sears Martha. <u>The Birth Book: Everything You Need to Know to Have a Safe and Satisfying Birth</u>. Little, Brown & Company. 1994. New York, NY.

Sekhavat et al. *The effects of Meperidine analgesia during labor on fetal heart rate.* International Journal of Biomedical Science. March 1, 2009. pg 59-61

Simkin, Penny. <u>Pregnancy, Childbirth, and the Newborn: The Complete Guide</u>. Meadowbrook Press, 2001 Minnetonka, MN.

Simonds, Wendy, Rothman, Barbara K., Norman, Bari M. <u>Laboring on: Birth in Transition in the United States.</u> Routledge, 2007. New York, NY.

Shapiro, Gottman, et al. *The baby and the marriage: Identifying factors that buffer against decline in marital satisfaction after the first baby arrives.* Journal of Family Psychology. Vol 14(1), Mar 2000, 59-70

Smolin & Grosvenor. <u>Nutrition Science and Applications</u>. John Wiley and Sons. 2003. Hoboken, N.J.

St. John Elaine, et al. *Hemorrhagic Disease of Newborn.* Med Scape emedicine. June 16, 2006

Stephenson, Rebecca G. and O'Connor, Linda J. <u>Obstetric and Gynecologic Care in Physical Therapy</u>, 2E. Slack Incorporated. 2000. New York, NY.